Permanent Disquiet

Permanent Disquiet: Psychoanalysis and the Transitional Subject comprises the second English language translation of some of Michel Émile de M'Uzan's key writings, alongside an invaluable glossary by Murielle Gagnebin of de M'Uzan's work. Together, they give a thorough overview of his key thinking.

The first part of the book sees de M'Uzan exploring the compatibility between creativity (particularly creative writing) and psychoanalytic practice and includes an exchange with Jean-Bertrand Pontalis. The second part focuses on de M'Uzan's key psychoanalytic concept – "permanent disquiet". Freud stated that the purpose of psychoanalysis was to transform neurotic suffering into common unhappiness. De M'Uzan built on this idea in his career and examined what it means for the clinical process for the analyst to step back, not to try and force happiness onto the patient, but instead to accept and allow them to find for themselves their own state of "permanent disquiet". Drawing on Freud and Winnicott and including an invaluable glossary of de M'Uzan's own psychoanalytic terms, this book brings de M'Uzan's powerful theory to the anglophone psychoanalytic world for the first time.

Permanent Disquiet: Psychoanalysis and the Transitional Subject will appeal to psychoanalysts and psychoanalytic psychotherapists globally who are interested in French psychoanalytic thought.

Michel Émile de M'Uzan (1921–2018) was a French neuropsychiatrist and psychoanalyst and founding member of the School of Psychosomatics of Paris, France (IPSO).

Recent titles in the Series include

The Analytical Process: Journeys and Pathways
Thierry Bokanowski

Psychotic Organisation of the Personality: Psychoanalytic Keys
Antonio Perez-Sanchez

Psychoanalytic Perspectives on Virtual Intimacy and Communication in Film
Edited by Andrea Sabbadini, Ilany Kogan and Paola Golinelli

Transformational Processes in Clinical Psychoanalysis: Dreaming, Emotions and the Present Moment
Lawrence J. Brown

The Psychoanalyst and the Child: From the consultation to psychoanalytic treatment
Michel Ody

Psychoanalytic Studies on Dysphoria: The False Accord in the Divine Symphony
Marion M. Oliner

Contemporary Perspectives on the Freudian Death Drive: In Theory, Clinical Practice and Culture
Edited by Victor Blüml, Liana Giorgi and Daru Huppert

Permanent Disquiet: Psychoanalysis and the Transitional Subject
Michel Émile de M'Uzan

For a full list of titles in this series, please visit www.routledge.com

Permanent Disquiet

Psychoanalysis and the Transitional Subject

Michel Émile de M'Uzan

With a glossary by Murielle Gagnebin of the principal notions developed by the author

Routledge
Taylor & Francis Group
LONDON AND NEW YORK

First published 2019
by Routledge
2 Park Square, Milton Park, Abingdon, Oxon OX14 4RN

and by Routledge
52 Vanderbilt Avenue, New York, NY 10017

Routledge is an imprint of the Taylor & Francis Group, an informa business

This book is a translation of a work previously published in French by Editions Gallimard as *L'inquiétude permanente: Suivi de Glossaire des principales notions élaborées par l'auteur* (2015).

Translated by Andrew Weller.

British Library Cataloguing-in-Publication Data
A catalogue record for this book is available from the British Library

Library of Congress Cataloging-in-Publication Data
A catalog record for this book has been requested

ISBN: 978-0-367-19366-9 (hbk)
ISBN: 978-0-367-19367-6 (pbk)
ISBN: 978-0-429-20195-0 (ebk)

Typeset in Palatino
by Apex CoVantage, LLC

Contents

Series editor's foreword

The Publications Committee of the International Psychoanalytic Association continues, with the present volume, the series "Psychoanalytic Ideas and Applications".

The aim of this series is to focus on the work of significant authors, whose works are outstanding contributions to the development of the psychoanalytic field. In doing so, this series will bring forward relevant ideas and themes, generated during the history of psychoanalysis, that deserve to be known and discussed by present-day psychoanalysts.

The relationship between psychoanalytic ideas and their applications needs to be put forward from the perspective of theory, clinical practice and research, in order to maintain their validity for contemporary psychoanalysis. The Publications Committee's objective is to share these ideas with the psychoanalytic community and with professionals in other related disciplines, so as to expand their knowledge and generate a productive interchange between the text and the reader.

The Publications Committee is proud to publish the translation of Michel Émile de M'Uzan's last book *Permanent Disquiet* (*L'Inquiétude permanente*). The English translation of this important volume clearly contributes to the Publications Committee's goal to make accessible crucial psychoanalytic contributions, in this case, from one of the most influential French psychoanalysts of the last half century. In this way, new bridges and dialogues amongst different psychoanalytic cultures can be established, enriching psychoanalytic theory and practice.

One of de M'Uzan's central interests dating back to his early publications has been the question of the uncertain nature of human identity. In this book, this topic is addressed through the theme of "permanent disquiet" (*l'inquiétude permanente*). The reader will find here his final contributions on the subject in which he expands and refines his views.

The reader unfamiliar with de M'Uzan's thinking will be intrigued by his ideas on the essence of psychoanalytic work and its goals. Differing from psychoanalytic perspectives in which the aim is to help the patient gain control of his or her instinctual life, allowing simultaneously a satisfaction acceptable to reality, de M'Uzan proposes that, in order to create an openness in the psychic functioning of the mind, it is necessary to disturb the illusion of uniqueness experienced by the subject. The analysand's experience of his or her identity achieved through the analytic process must reach a state of vacillation where the frontiers between ego and non-ego are experienced as indeterminate (attaining a sense of permanent disquiet). It is in this state, de M'Uzan believes, that changes in the patient's psychic life can take place. By expanding the subject's identity, psychoanalysis enriches and broadens the subjective experience. The permanent disquiet is not, therefore, a strategical goal of analysis, but the effect of it, a consequence of a greater openness to one's self.

In addition to the chapters dedicated to the topic of identity, the reader will also find fictional short stories written by de M'Uzan as well as a glossary of the principal notions developed by the author, which has been put together by Murielle Gagnebin. De M'Uzan noted that the glossary "shows simultaneously the architecture of my thinking, its development and its continuity".

I have no doubt that this book is a great contribution. The English translation of this important volume makes accessible to the broad psychoanalytic readership one of the most important contributions on the topic of identity in the psychoanalytic literature.

Gabriela Legorreta
Series Editor
Chair, IPA Publications Committee

Preface

To suggest that at the end of a well-conducted analysis the analysand emerges with a "permanent disquiet"* may seem counterintuitive if not outright bad publicity for psychoanalysis. Does it not appear as if the author was advertising negative results? Well, it depends on how you conceive psychoanalysis. In a way, this sort of problem was addressed early on by Freud himself when he seriously, but not without humour, stated that the goal of psychoanalysis is to transform neurotic suffering into common unhappiness. Freud's remark has been traditionally put on the account of his tragic outlook on existence, but it could just as well be ascribed to a radical truthfulness on his part, regarding both the practical possibilities *and* the very Ethics of psychoanalysis.

Psychoanalysis never promised happiness, not only because its method of treatment – no more than any other – could not achieve such an outcome, but also, and perhaps more importantly, because pursuing that sort of result constitutes a serious breach in the ethical stance required of anyone who intends to practice psychoanalysis. Obviously, one wishes that the analysand will in the end have a better life; this can be formulated using an economic point of view: it is a matter of "[putting] psychic energy back into circulation where it has been immobilized by the regime of binding" (p. 122 of this volume). But this is no recipe for happiness, whatever that word may mean. It is a matter of gaining or regaining the often quoted capacity to love and to work, i.e. of being able to put psychic energy to good use. But there is another aspect to this. As is well known, Freud recommended that during the session the analyst entertain no particular purposive idea or, more literally, no goal-representation (*Zielvorstellung*).[1] This also is a principle not due to Freud's personal idiosyncrasy, but which is part of the fundamental rule to be followed for anyone who wishes to truly listen to the other – i.e. without superimposing one's own expectations or preferences – and to favour the emergence of the repressed. It is certainly a radical requirement, one that every analyst soon finds quite difficult to fulfil. But such incomplete fulfilment is no excuse for not trying. It is indeed amidst the tension created between our natural goal-seeking tendency and the ideal of pursuing no goal in particular that the resistance of the analyst will become observable. Such resistance, it must be added, matters just as much as the analysand's resistance and both constitute our best guides towards discovering the unconscious.

It is therefore a matter of ethical integrity on the part of the analyst when Michel Émile de M'Uzan's proposes that analysis is conducive not to serenity or happiness, but to some "enduring concern" (another possible translation of *"l'inquiétude permanente"*). But wait! Isn't *this* a specific goal entertained by de M'Uzan? Not really, if we consider that the permanent disquiet he alludes to is a *result* of analysis, not an objective to be actively pursued. In plain words, it entails acknowledging what the psychoanalytic investigation of the personality teaches: notably, that there is no single identity and that the analysand may discover what Rimbaud had beautifully formulated: "I is another" (*Je est un autre* – see p. xiii), i.e. we are all endowed with a *spectrum of identity*,* or, as de M'Uzan also writes, we are *transitional subjects*.* The concern implied in the permanent disquiet is not at all reducible to worry or anxiety; it is a concern and a sense of care for oneself and for the other – the other in the outside world and the otherness within. Though not a goal purposefully pursued by the analyst, the greater flexibility or malleability that the analysand may reach through the process of analysis will reveal itself a most desirable result. It is de M'Uzan's version of what Freud possibly meant when, in the later part of his writings, he stated that a general result of psychoanalysis should be that *"Where Id was, there Ego shall be"* (Freud, 1933, p. 80). This formula has often been interpreted as meaning that the ego should *replace* the id. But a close reading could also show it to mean that the ego of the subject emerging from analysis feels more at ease in its relationship to the id, that it can dwell in id territory without raising rigid defensive barriers; in other words, it can more easily deal with the otherness within. De M'Uzan formulates this in a most radical way: *"Where Ego is, there Id shall be"* (see p. 116).

So this is no state of bliss. The drives that constitute the id remain unchanged, and they keep challenging the ego's desire for undisturbed quietness. What is changed, however, is that the subject is now more capable not only of facing the turbulence brought about by the id, but more importantly, of making use of such disturbance for reconfiguring, time and again, its own spectrum of identity. More porous barriers – i.e. more flexible and uncertain ego limits resulting from the analytic process – are not liabilities, but assets that contribute to a richer capacity to meet a fellow human being as well as to transform one's own drive impulses into creative endeavours.

The closeness to some of Winnicott's views is here apparent, though the differences should not be glossed over. Whereas Winnicott (1971) was interested in transitional space, objects and phenomena, de M'Uzan concentrates on the *transitional subject*.* In a way, this is well in line with

Winnicott, but it also represents a more radical take. Whereas Winnicott speaks of the Self, including in terms of true and false Self, the concept of Self was not, to my knowledge, critically examined by him. At the risk of overly simplifying, one could say that in Winnicott's view the Self is expected to be more integrated and strengthened by the work of analysis, and this is certainly somehow desirable. One must ponder, however, what the notion of "integration" implies. I believe that in de M'Uzan's view, integration does not in the least suggest a more "unified" Self; integration, if de M'Uzan were to use that term in relation to the subject, would rather mean – and this may well be implicit in Winnicott as well – the coexistence of different but dynamically balanced elements. By "dynamically balanced" I mean: in constant renegotiation of their compatibility. Stated differently, *the transitional subject encompasses both identity and otherness*, and there is no single or monolithic identity; there is always a double and even, as mentioned earlier, a *spectrum* of identity, without any notion of "falseness" implied. Interestingly, however, if we think that Winnicott's "false self" was also dubbed by him the "caretaker self" (Abram, 1996, p. 304), then it has indeed some resemblance with de M'Uzan's *double*, especially as the latter comes to the rescue, so to speak, in situations of extreme psychical or physical danger, terminal illness, imminent death and so on. Except that the double in de M'Uzan's view has nothing false about it, nor does it present itself first (as Winnicott's false self is supposed to do); the double usually works in the background, only to emerge in situations of apparently unsolvable contradictions.[2]

***

Readers of *Death and Identity*, de M'Uzan's (2013b) previous book in English, may have become somewhat acquainted with the array of original concepts that were introduced by de M'Uzan in the course of his long career. For them and those for whom this is a first acquaintance, the present book contains a precious tool: Murielle Gagnebin's glossary. A very useful instrument indeed, as it not only lists the series of concepts and gives a thorough definition for each of them, but also provides cross-references to the major texts where the concepts appear. The reader is thus enabled to get a wider view of de M'Uzan's psychoanalytic landscape. De M'Uzan was Murielle Gagnebin's companion in life so her contribution to the book was constantly discussed and validated by her late husband. Thanks to this glossary, one can get even more familiar with de M'Uzan's thinking and with the truly original set of conceptual tools forming the armature of this bold clinical and theoretical body of knowledge.

***

De M'Uzan left us at the beginning of 2018. Until the end, he remained one of, if not *the*, most respected French psychoanalyst. To those who had the good luck of knowing him personally, his kindness, charm and sense of humour were unequalled. His clinical and theoretical thoroughness, coupled with his deep originality, will be certainly missed. It is my hope that by making available yet another important set of his papers to an English-language readership, this book will help his unique contribution to psychoanalysis live on.

Dominique Scarfone

Notes

1 Bion (1970) formulated the same idea by advocating for the analyst the "suspension of memory, desire and understanding" (p. 43).
2 I have contributed a personal example in my Preface to de M'Uzan's previous book in English, *Death and Identity* (de M'Uzan, 2013, p. xi).

References

Abram, Jan (1996). *The language of Winnicott: A dictionary of Winnicott's use of words.* London: Clunie Press.
Bion, Wilfred Ruprecht (1970). *Attention and interpretation: A scientific approach to insight in psycho-analysis and groups.* London: Tavistock.
de M'Uzan, Michel (2013). *Death and identity: Being and the psycho-sexual drama.* (trans. Andrew Weller), London: Karnac Books.
Freud, Sigmund (1933a). *New introductory lectures on psycho-analysis.* The Standard Edition of the Complete Psychological Works of Sigmund Freud, Vol XXII (1932–1936), London, The Hogarth Press and the Institute of Psychoanalysis.
Winnicott, D. W. (1971). Transitional objects and Transitional Phenomena, In *Playing and Reality*. London: Tavistock Publications.

Foreword

In the exchange that we had a long time ago of which I will only give a few fragments here, J.-B. Pontalis saw no obstacle to the compatibility between the writing of fiction and analytic practice (de M'Uzan & Pontalis, 1977) – something his literary work showed so well. For my part, although I was the author of three books of "short stories" (de M'Uzan, 1954, 1962, 1994a), I did not think this was really possible and I argued that the pervasive impact of the living – the impact of the patient – invaded one's whole mind and made the daily exercise of writing fiction difficult to reconcile with analytic practice, especially as it has the tendency to take hold of one's thinking fraudulently. Several articles linked to this theme that were published between 2005 and 2015 have been brought together here in the first part under the title "Artists and their hell".

The second part of this book is organised around the theme of "permanent disquiet"*[1] which, for me, is the true aim of analysis. This disquiet, as Murielle Gagnebin points out in her glossary, is the result of a "scandal of identity"* that must be triggered or aggravated during analysis. It is a matter of intervening in a self-preservative *field of identity*, that is to say, non-sexual and thus not drive-related. Consequently, it is important to disturb, disorganise and undo, as a point of reference, what Phyllis Greenacre (1958) has famously described as the sense of uniqueness experienced by an integrated organism that is able to recognise others without ambiguity. When we have in mind the most authentic aspects of a human being, the liberation of what is most personal about him or her, it is a matter of guaranteeing the subject the possibility of attaining a state of "permanent disquiet",* that is to say, of coming to the point at which the uncertain and aleatory character of being must be discovered as a fundamental fact. "I" ("*Je*") must be able to recognise itself as the other, but rather differently from how Rimbaud had supposed:

> I witness the unfolding of my thought: I watch it, I listen to it: I make a stroke of the bow: the symphony makes its stir in the depths of the pit or comes in one leap on to the stage.
>
> (*Correspondances* [Letter dated 15 May 1871 to Paul Demeny] in Rimbaud, 1972, p. 249)

In effect, while Rimbaud claimed to be a "seer" and hoped "to arrive at the unknown by the dissoluteness of *all the senses*" (*Correspondances* [Letter dated 15 May 1871 to George Ibamzard] in Rimbaud, 1972, p. 248), I am referring to a "psychological chimera"* that designates a sort of new organism arising from the meeting of two unconscious minds, that of the analysand and that of his or her analyst. It is a monster possessing its own modes of functioning. The growth of this fabulous child is affected by various influences from its creators. There are those that are related to the analysand's structure. But we must also take into account those that depend on the analyst and which proceed from a special disposition for primary identification and a tolerance for experiences of "depersonalisation".* I also have in mind my "spectrum of identity",* a zone where the frontiers between ego and non-ego are more than indeterminate, and whose constitution attests, in both protagonists, to a disposition for primary identification which allows the chimera to come into being. The idea of a "dissolution of frontiers", of "imbrication", is no longer sufficient for me: it is a matter, certainly, of an "essential feature of being" in accordance with the discoveries of biology for which the frontier between the inert and the living is unstable and uncertain. I adopt as a fundamental notion the "science of indefinite limits". And I would add that "we will have to accept that beyond its therapeutic project, psychoanalysis . . . gives access to a sense of 'permanent disquiet'"* (see de M'Uzan, 2009, p. 97; 2013b, p. 200; 2011b, p. 31).

The third part is comprised of a glossary that is very important in my view. I have, in fact, often given literary titles to my writings, which does not allow the reader to find the notions that I have introduced or the different use that I have made of certain others that are in usage. Concerning the fifty notions that make up this glossary, after each entry the original text in which the notion was "coined" is given, and then the book in which one can find it, followed by other texts which prepare, or sometimes foreshadow the arrival of other notions that shed light on it retrospectively. Alongside these "notions" – I prefer the term notion to that of concept, which is too clear cut – the reader will find "classical" notions such as the "death drive",* for example, against which I have fought, in an attempt to restore dignity to Freud's systemic unconscious. I explain in it my reasons for not retaining these terms which, in my view, are unsuited to Freud's own authentic thought, and psychoanalytic thought in general. The reader will also find in this glossary my discussions with certain psychoanalysts who had more or less adopted a particular expression – which shows that it was good! – while making a different use of it. I had to clarify things. This was the case, for example, of my "psychological chimera" (de M'Uzan, 1978).

This glossary shows simultaneously the architecture of my thinking, its developments and its continuity. From the outset my patients seem to have brought me the material which would permit me, bit by bit, to forge a new psychoanalytic theory. This vigilant glossary was entirely established by Murielle Gagnebin, but it is a text written, as it were, with four hands.

Note

1 The words and expressions followed by an asterisk are defined in the glossary.

Part I

Artists and their hell

Chapter 1

Interview with J.-B. Pontalis (fragments) (1977)[1]

The central theme of this exchange of views raises several questions related to the transition from analytic practice to theoretical writing (that of the *écrivant*, as Roland Barthes[2] would have said), and, furthermore, highlights the problems of compatibility between the profession of the psychoanalyst and that of the writer. In the pages preceding these extracts, J.-B. Pontalis calls into question the general view of a priority of what is experienced over what is thought and of what is thought (*le pensé*) over what is written (*l'écrit*). For him, the movement of analysis is one that goes, on the contrary, from "words to the flesh". The writing of the analyst would no longer be seen, then, "as a defence against analytic experience; it would become almost an integral part of it". This relationship, which he considers to be very intimate, is lived out, however, in a state of "relative *competition*" and "relative *incompatibility*". In my view, however, although the authentic writer has nothing to fear from lying on the couch, the rivalry between the writing of fiction which is the true purpose of the writer and analytic practice seems to me to be a radical obstacle.

MICHEL ÉMILE DE M'UZAN The writer, and the artist in general, has nothing to fear from analysis, the experience of which is in no way sterilising, contrary to the prejudice that you have just mentioned. I have been able to observe this myself more than once, like many other analysts. Freud, the very first analyst, asserted in a letter that when the impulse to create is stronger than the inner resistances, analysis can only increase, not diminish the creative faculties. This concurs, moreover, with my experience. Artists – whatever form their apprehension may take – often come to analysis when they feel blocked in their work. We know that this is only an argument that allows them to take the initial step, just as the desire for analytic training covers the deep motivations of the future analyst. It remains true, however, that it is to be hoped that analysis removes the inhibitions of the artist and, generally speaking, this is what happens.

J.-B. PONTALIS *My experience confirms yours. But as these inhibitions cannot be considered as a symptom isolated from the mind as a whole, this is a sign that literature and psychoanalysis are not mutually exclusive. Unless you consider, that is, and this is another proposition that is often put forward, that analyses of writers do not go as "far" as others, leaving, by common agreement, a remainder?*

M. – It is very difficult to give you an answer to that. However, I would venture to say that I do not see what, in practical terms, prevents the analysis of a writer from being taken as far as any other. We could certainly discuss this from a theoretical angle, but in practice, in the reality of analytic treatments, I cannot see what could prevent this. Not only can a writer consult an analyst for personal difficulties as much as for difficulties related to work, but we can sometimes observe the emergence of a desire to write in the course of an analysis in someone who previously had never thought of doing so, for his or her project was quite different.

P. – *That does not, however, make a writer.*

M. – When I speak of the emergence of a desire to write – of a need to write – I am thinking of one that leads to an authentic realisation and that may be recognised by others. I have followed analysands who previously had no experience of personal literary activity, in whom the analysis freed up creative capacities in this domain, capacities that were expressed subsequently in a continuous and efficient manner – and not episodically or in a purely defensive mode. This will not come as a surprise to the analyst who is used to seeing new forms of creativity develop in their patients in one domain or another. Let me repeat: I cannot see any radical incompatibility between the fact of pursuing one's analysis as far as possible and the fact of writing – or of painting – etc. If there is any incompatibility – since this is the issue we are discussing – it is not between personal analysis and writing, but between the practice of analysis as an analyst and a genuine activity as a writer. It seems to me that there are deep reasons for this. I would not claim to be able to enumerate them, and even less to be able to elucidate them. For the time being, I would just like to mention one of them. Forgive me for being schematic, but in doing so I will perhaps be clearer. Whatever may be said about it, the movement of analysis is, in certain respects, reductive. Indeed, this is precisely one of the criticisms that is often made of analysis – a criticism that has some validity, no doubt, and I am exposing myself to it – since analysts hardly ever fail to defend themselves against this accusation. They are wrong in doing so, for the notion of a reductive movement is essential, innovative and even inspired in that it invites us to look towards the "bottom" (*le "bas"*) and to cease to make the overly sublime "top" (*le "haut"*) – even cultural – the primary agent of "creative activities". The movement of analysis goes from the complex to the elementary, to the vulgar; in a certain way, it simplifies. Through interpretation,* analysis renders the meaning of abundant and complex manifest contents, revealing the simple and raw latent meaning in a secondarised formulation that employs direct language. This is certainly a very ordinary idea, but one that has its place because it defines a directly opposite movement to that of the creative process, at any rate in the literary domain we are discussing. Let me add that I am thinking precisely of the writing of fiction, whether a story or a poem, which I distinguish clearly from criticism.

. . .

I am setting aside the category of writings that is called, I think, "moved" criticism, where the aesthetic dimension is particularly present, and whose power depends on its noticeable rootedness in a nocturnal, and perhaps wild, universe. Critical writings, in the strict sense of the term, seem for their part to be oriented initially by a desire for demonstration, a line of argumentation whose logic might be found in very different domains. Admittedly, it is sometimes the case that one is both a critic and a writer of fiction. But this is not the common run of things.

P. – *All the same for Baudelaire, Henry James and Proust, just to mention a few authors, literature, you would not disagree, I think, was their passion, their life. . . . But let us return to the opposition that you insist on between practising analysis and the activity of a writer.*

M. – My point is that the driving forces behind each of them are exactly converse. In a piece of fictional writing, we are not going in the direction of decoding but, on the contrary, in the direction of a proliferation of what is manifest, where the language used seems to be marked by a sort of formal regression in which the figures become increasingly symbolic before constituting a series of masks. Basically, writing consists in saying while not saying, in saying something other than what one thinks one is saying, in lying without knowing it in order to reveal some ignored truth. The writer is constantly showing and hiding, and the succession of masks that he constructs give his writing the striking character that discursive language does not possess.

P. – *I agree with what you say about the writer: he says without saying, he conceals as much as he shows, etc. . . . Confusing interpretation with decoding would perhaps be true for those Kleinians who carry their dictionary around with them in their heads. But when the analyst refuses this easy option, when he does not treat interpretation as simultaneous translation, when he does not consider himself as the holder of a set of keys that will open all doors – and, in my view, close them – what happens? The analyst is then not only led to listen to the latent content of the statements and silences of his patient, but also to be receptive to his own latent contents, to what the analysand induces in him. You yourself have shown how this highly singular communication between the patient and the analyst occurs. I am thinking in particular of your text on the "paradoxical countertransference". This way of seeing things has even been reproached for being too risky, too subjective. . . .*

M. – That's true.

P. – *There is, then, a trajectory operating in analysis that is not very different from that which motivates the writer. For the writer is not only in search of what he is unaware of, of the unknown in himself; he also seeks to generate a similar movement in the reader. The reader, like the author, is only interested in what is "manifest", at least during the time of reading, which ultimately is the only one that matters. It is only secondarily, by stepping back, that he will fall back on his own code and become a critic-interpreter. But, as I said at the outset, reading, for me, is not interpreting; it is more a question of regressing with everything positive that that involves.*

M. – You have just introduced a further element, or rather an additional character: the reader. I was considering one character only, namely, the analyst who is pursuing side by side his activities as a practitioner and as a writer. The opposition that I have made between the two functions is admittedly a bit too clear cut because the analyst may have a "literary" ear for the discourse of his patient – which, to my mind, is not pejorative – linked to this very particular countertransference, the essence of which is very close to that which nurtures the inspiration of the writer or the dreamer. The two universes are thus not fundamentally heterogeneous; I think I have explained myself sufficiently on this point elsewhere (de M'Uzan, 1977). I would add that it is certainly not a matter of chance if analysts have taken so much interest in literature. They felt they were directly concerned. No, what I have in mind is, on the one hand, the movement of the action that orients both activities, its direction, and, on the other, the specific characteristics of the psychic economy of the analyst and of the writer. Irrespective of the relative uncertainty or indefiniteness of the frontiers between the subject and his objects – and you know how much I am attached to this idea – the analyst is essentially oriented, polarised, and sometimes even invaded, by the discourse of another person. Being able to allow himself to be pervaded by this extraneous discourse is indeed one of the qualities that the analyst should possess. The movement that sustains the writer goes in exactly the opposite direction. Basically, the writer turns towards himself while inducing – sometimes artificially – a real regression. The work he does subsequently on the ideational contents arising from this regression occurs according to specific laws, in particular those of written language. You will tell me that the analyst also regresses during the session, with his patient, something with which I am, of course, in complete agreement. But we do not know, first of all, to whom the "partial ideational contents" mobilised by this regression belong and, furthermore, they are dealt with quite differently. The requirements of their formation, of their potential verbalisation, are also original; they do not have the same cultural reference points, at least not exactly, quite apart from the fact that they have others. Furthermore, the laws that govern their formulation, their grammar,* as it were, are in the service of a clarification, of an elucidation. When all things are said and done, I make a clear distinction between the work carried out in relation to the discourse of another person and that which pertains to the figures emerging from an inner proliferation of activity.

The other aspect of this opposition between the analyst and the writer that I am trying to circumscribe – even excessively, as a tactic – has to do with the economy of the two activities. For me, the writer is someone whose first and primordial task is writing. It is writing that gives a decisive direction to his days and which constitutes his essential investment. Any other activity – however much time he devotes objectively to writing, but generally speaking it is a great deal – is experienced as secondary or accessory; in certain respects it is devalued, or even, in extreme situations, scorned. The writer, as we know, is quick to complain when these tasks – life, in short, "take" up his time, time with which he will perhaps do nothing. This is how, in part, the very particular status of his narcissism is expressed, and the meaning of his life defined. Something Arthur Adamov[3] said to me one day comes to mind here: "When one writes, it's terrifying; when one doesn't write, it's horrific".

. . .

What I have in mind is the depth, the seriousness of the commitment, the importance that the writer ascribes to his non-literary activities. Even more than the time he devotes objectively to writing, what counts is what, qualitatively speaking, he puts of himself both into his writing and into his other occupations. This being so, it remains true overall, "musings" included – and we know how important they are – that the qualitative distribution of interests tends to follow this movement. There are not many of whom it could be said that their life is that of a writer, since they devote most of themselves to some other task.

P. – *Someone who writes a book, doesn't that exist for you?*

M. – Indeed. One book, even if it is sublime, does not make a writer. This book will perhaps have its place in literary history – although when it is a one-off, its fate is very uncertain. In this precise case, can we say that the author of this book was still a writer when his footsteps took him elsewhere, that he was living in another universe? Think of the case of Rimbaud.

P. – *And you, for your part, do not forget* "The Princess of Cleves." . . .[4] *That said, let us try to clarify what differentiates our respective points of view. I agree with you in recognising that one cannot, at one and the same time, be an analyst and a writer, and in accepting the fact that one cannot, at the end of one's day of doing analysis, find in oneself the inner resources necessary for nourishing the work of a writer. One is not "in the right condition". But that is simply observing a fact, namely, the question of psychic economy at a given time, which doesn't take us very far.*

M. – Absolutely, yes.

P. – *You will accept that it is not only the possibility of writing that is then excluded. The analyst is also often not very available for other commitments that would mobilize him deeply; indeed, his loved ones sometimes reproach him for this. . . . Without wishing to fall further into the pathos of "the analyst's being", let us recognise that analytic asceticism cuts us off somewhat – like the writer, in your understanding of the word, moreover – from the outside world. We are not always easy to live with. . . .*

M. – Let's say that, in other circumstances, there is nothing to stop an analyst who no longer practices for one reason or another, or very little, from writing or taking up writing again. It is a question, in fact, of psychic economy: when an analyst's interest and energy have been mobilised by patients, by others, he is no longer available for himself. But alongside this question of psychic economy, and linked with it, there is this movement of the analytic work of which I was speaking earlier, which develops in a direction that is exactly opposite to that of writing. This I continue to maintain, even if you corrected, quite rightly, my somewhat schematic formulations, for while the analyst and the writer have the same basic material in common, they have a different way of dealing with it. Do you believe that, from one moment to another, one can "turn the switch" and adopt an entirely different mode of functioning? The analyst may take pleasure, somewhat perversely, in immerging himself in a stream of bizarre images without knowing any longer whether they concern him or his patient, while the language of the protagonists, at certain moments, makes use of uncontrolled archaic means. The analyst may then think he is a poet, and even be capable of making puns! But this only lasts for a short time. It may certainly be a fruitful phase, but it cannot last because it is necessary to extricate oneself from this humus before getting bogged down in it, and to return, whether one likes it or not, to lucidity.

The writer, for his part, does not want to understand. He uses writing to complicate everything. From a mere meander he creates an inextricable maze from which new paths are constantly emerging that fascinate and mislead. In this way, as I was saying, he is forever creating masks that overlap each other.

P. – *I see now how our views of literature, and perhaps also of psychoanalysis, are not exactly the same. Yes, literary fiction is a maze. But in the labyrinth, one has a rendezvous with the, with one's, Minotaur. And one also sometimes has the possibility of holding Ariadne's thread in one's hand! Put another way, in fiction, truth is not absent. And conversely, in analysis, the work of truth only takes place through a series of masks. The analyst does not possess his patient's truth. An interpretation proposed as "true" today will appear "false" tomorrow. In our own way, we are constructing a novel. The truth, for us, is not a thing, but a work, a movement. It wants to say, but it doesn't say. . . .*

M. – The truth, that is a very equivocal subject. I once suggested that what is "beautiful" might well only be what is "true", although, almost in the same breath, I saw the lie as one of the essential motive forces of writing. Singing the praises of lies will not come as too much of a surprise, perhaps, if we recognise that a story, precisely, is made up of a series of disguises of which the writer is far from being the master. One writes because one cannot do otherwise. There is no real freedom. Writing is sometimes the best or the only means some people have of dealing with the demands of their psychic economy. As for the quest for truth (which truth?), I would not say that it is absent, but that it manifests itself above all at the technical level. And if it were only a matter of "finding" the word or the phrase, the construction that would win over the reader would convince him, even while deceiving him.

P. – *Let's try to get beyond the level of generalities. After all, we have both been personally interested, for different reasons, by the articulation and the rupture between writing and psychoanalysing. You wrote fiction before being an analyst, didn't you?*

M. – Indeed, for me writing came well before analysis. I mean that I had begun to write well before I discovered a specific interest in analysis, and particularly before I had any desire to become an analyst. Subsequently

I thought that the writer could continue to write and pursue analytic practice at the same time. I even saw analysis as the agent of a reconciliation between life and writing which seemed to me, in certain respects, to be outside life. What I meant by life, very simply, was the world of action, for example, practising medicine or teaching. Analysis was also life but, at the same time, something quite different. I pointed out earlier, did I not, that analysis and literature shared practically the same material? So I believed analysis, which I did not in any way regard as compromise, would permit life to intervene without going against the current of literature.

P. – *So, at that moment you saw yourself continuing to write, while practising analysis?*

M. – Yes.

P. – *Without any discordance?*

M. – I did not consider the possibility of any discordance; quite the contrary. In fact, the beginning of my interest in psychoanalysis and, above all, personal analysis, was the agent of a significant movement in favour of writing. Through it I discovered a sort of new creative impulse, perhaps even a fresh vigour that I didn't have before.

P. – *Your personal experience of analysis anticipated what you saw confirmed later, when you had writers in treatment with you.*

M. – Absolutely.

P. – *It was more of a fresh stimulus, then, than a blockage.*

M. – Unquestionably. Subsequently, it was my involvement in the "analytic career" that gradually oriented me differently. One day, I realised that I was writing less and less (I mean tales or short stories). It was not that I was questioning what I was still writing more than before. No new factor was involved in criticising negatively these recent productions. It simply happened that I was no longer a writer, even though I still sometimes wrote.

P. – *Fiction?*

M. – Yes. At the moment, writing, at least in the sense in which I understand it, is far from being at the centre of my concerns. It may be that this will turn out to be a transitory period. This possibility needs to be preserved, even when I am speaking of a prolonged present. Writing would then be a potential activity, as evidenced by the incessant emergence in me of unquestionably literary themes, themes, therefore, that only literature could develop. But that is not what writing is. When writing is an essential investment, one begins one's days by writing. The rest comes afterwards. It may be that this attitude is the fruit of a monstrous error – yet another lie. But that is how it is. First one works, that is writing. Afterwards, it is something else.

P. – *What brought about this change, do you think?*

M. – It was the practice of analysis. Practising analysis does not destroy the literary material, as one often hears. But it engenders a "diversion" of activity. For me, what I was activating, whenever I wrote, was literarily just as satisfying, and even "better", than what I had been able to do before. But I insist, there is an enormous difference between the status of the writer and that of the analyst who sometimes writes, irrespective of the value of his writings.

What could I add to explain my evolution? I would be tempted to make the analysands responsible, which is perhaps a way of fooling myself. The fact is that their presence is extraordinarily imperious. They drain the major part of one's interest. The horizon is the session and not the blank sheet of paper.

P. – *You could be a writer on holiday, on holiday from the transference, on holiday from this imperative?*

M. – On holiday from the countertransference. Do you think one has any control over that? Analysts take long holidays. And what do they write during them? Psychoanalysis, of course. But I would like to move on to another aspect of the problem. Very abruptly, and to be intentionally provocative, I would say that writing is useless! Writing is a vain activity. No one needs our books, whereas people do need analysis.

P. – *The unconscious is perhaps unaware of time, but psychoanalysis, for its part, belongs to history. Humanity did without it for centuries. And, as I was saying to you at the beginning of the interview, literature, to some degree, stood in for it. That is to say, literature, in our civilization; and elsewhere, myths. I would even say that the current difficulty in being a writer lies in the fact that a function that was formerly fulfilled quite naturally by literature is today more suspect and seems to be more vain, because psychoanalysis has taken over from it. A woman no longer looks for herself in* "Madame Bovary" *but in the "Case of Dora".*

But there are readers, fortunately, because otherwise there would no longer be any literature. "Nourishing oneself on books" can, at least in certain phases of existence, be something vital. I am suspicious of the conjunction nowadays of two attitudes that are only apparently contradictory: "Culture", offered as a consumer product – and yet, nourishing oneself is not about consuming anything, anyhow, one does not look at a painting in a supermarket – and by the same token the disdain for literature, the rejection of the notion of oeuvre, the rotating stand replacing the bookshop and, worse still, the whirlpool of ideas – one fad per season – which seeks to impose itself as a new way of thinking. Of course, the world can do very well without literature but, as Sartre once said, it can do without man even better. . . . Everything would then function without any difficulty.

M. – If in that sense literature is doubtful, analytic activity, for its part, is indubitable. Although it is somewhat fashionable to say the contrary, this function justifies itself, as it were, naturally. There's no question about it. The writer, on the other hand, in his troubled subjectivity, must legitimise his art, create its justification. And this he must do day after day. It is only through his daily work, with its share of troubles – for one does not write as a bird sings – that the writer convinces himself of the self-evidence of his activity, that he accepts that it exists by right. This situation is perhaps part of the inner drama of the artist. . . . But the public, more often than not, knows nothing of it.

P. – *But this self-evidence that you recognise in analysis, this sense of uncertainty and of perpetually starting over and over again that you ascribe to literature, do they not reside simply in the fact that you "invest" in analysis completely and have ceased, relatively speaking, to invest in writing?*

. . .

M. – Let's be quite clear: analysis can only impose itself as self-evident when it truly constitutes a practice. Anyone who is satisfied with doing two or three sessions a day is not an analyst. For him, analysis simply does not exist . . . or doesn't exist any longer. Personal investment in analytic activity is certainly essential; but, in spite of everything, the latter sustains itself in a way that is more natural, it seems to me, than literary activity, more spontaneous, easier. I recognise that the doubt concerning the significance, the meaning, of writing only develops when a sort of initial naivety, no doubt shared by many, has been lost – and this happens very quickly. Thereafter, doubt is an intrinsic part of the activity of writing. The analyst, on the other hand, whatever his difficulties and questionings may be – and we know how heavily they can weigh on him – does not seem to me to feel to such a degree the need to justify the legitimacy of his activity. It can almost be taken for granted.

. . .

P. – *I think that analysis is justified by little more than itself. One could say of it – as of literature – that it is an "interminable aim". Admitting as much does not lead to scepticism or to disdain for the results. But the criterion of usefulness does not guide the analyst, in my opinion, any more than the writer. Self-evidence is neither more nor less natural or social in either case. All that counts is the quantity and the quality of the investment involved, for the analyst and his patient and for the writer and his reader alike.*

M. – But in saying that don't you think you are reducing the importance of the therapeutic implications of analysis? We both know that it is not fashionable to speak about it, but it remains true that these implications are part of the very definition of analysis, of the original definition that Freud gave of it. There is no doubt that therapeutic concerns are not, and cannot be, constantly present in our minds when we are listening to patients. This barely needs pointing out. Nevertheless, I remain convinced that, even at a latent level, this "idea" is never really evacuated: it is fundamentally active in us and gives a certain legitimacy to our activity. Moreover, this feature of self-evidence is also derived from the particularity that psychoanalysis offers as an organically constituted whole: that is to say, it is a way of understanding the functioning of psychic life and its disturbances; a technique for treating these disturbances; and an instrument of knowledge applied to the most diverse products of the thought of man and of his culture. This is what makes psychoanalysis a unique and incomparable science, different from all the others, none of which has integrated the dimension of the unconscious.

P. – *I agree with all that. But let's move on. We can see a bit more clearly now why one cannot be the servant of two equally demanding masters – literature and psychoanalysis – at the same time; unless one is called Harlequin.*

How then should psychoanalytic writing be considered? Should it be regarded as a compromise formation, as a symptom, or as the more or less satisfactory solution of a conflict between two movements or two vocations? Is there a point of reconciliation between the writer and the psychoanalyst here? Or is it the hybrid product of a failed writer and an accomplished psychoanalyst, unless – a more cruel but plausible hypothesis – analytic writing is the product of a double failure?

M. – I cannot see any relationship between a piece of analytic writing and a piece of fiction. For me, a piece of analytic writing is more akin to criticism, if only because the technique of writing employed is very similar. In analytic writing, thought is more in the background and becomes part of the flow of an essentially discursive linear development. Aesthetic concerns – words certainly raise many problems – are rather secondary. What matters first and foremost is to be clear and correct, which analysts who write a lot, too much perhaps, often forget.

In a piece of "fiction", critical distance does not operate at the same level, hence the frequent impasses that are literally constitutive of the work. The writer is engulfed by a world of egotistical, powerful and imperious ideas or images. And he must also extricate himself from this if he is to be able to carry out quite a different work, almost contrary, on words, on propositions. He must pursue this latter task, which connects him with a long cultural past, with history, with extreme rigour, something analytic writing does not require to the same degree.

P. – *If I think of your recent writings, of "S.j.e.m."* ("Si j'étais mort") *(de M'Uzan, 1974a), I find something that is very similar to a literary work. Admittedly, the concern for demonstration is present, but it is not the primary concern. What comes first is a very singular intuition or a sentence that imposed itself on you.*

M. – With regard to the text that you have just cited, I concede that I adopted a more literary point of view than is usually the case. This relative exception – and analytic literature presents many others – ought therefore to justify your position. And yet, I still maintain that the two genres are heterogeneous. In psychoanalytic writings related to literary texts, it remains a fact that the development of the text is organised with the aim of transmitting knowledge, an experience or a series of reflections on a given topic. Even if the manner is not strictly discursive, it is subject to the requirements of demonstration. In a literary text, the author always seems to me to be driven, sometimes unwittingly, by a need to decentre his reader, as he was himself at the beginning and at certain moments in his work. He seeks to attract the reader towards another world by depriving him of his usual points of reference. Ultimately, and without necessarily being conscious of it, he hopes, with entirely original means to shake up the common sense of a solid "delimitation of the body". You will no doubt tell me that a good many analysts are driven by a similar intention that is often very conscious. They are the ones, in general, who overvalue writing, and whose ambitions are perhaps first and foremost literary. This can be seen especially in France, where this or that analyst is no longer particularly concerned with transmitting something, but with having an effect on his reader, with attracting his attention more by means of formulations than ideas. And, as the analytic text is not well-suited to this way of proceeding, the undertaking, let me be quite frank, is inevitably a failure. It no longer even has the value of a compromise, the dignity of a symptom.

P. – *The undertaking might not be a failure if the analyst was also a writer.*

M. – In that case, if he wanted to decentre his reader, he would be more likely to write a story.

P. – *Agreed. . . .*

M. – I can perfectly well conceive of the case of an analyst who was capable of theorising in the context of a seminar, but who otherwise felt no need to write. Someone, that is, who had a vast amount of knowledge and a deep capacity for theoretical reflection, but who was not concerned by writing. After all, we do not always use in a text the product of our musings about theory or about our practice. These musings which occur unexpectedly, sometimes when we are out walking, are nonetheless just as fruitful, if not more so, than our laborious reflections at our work table, and yet we allow them to slip through our fingers. That at least is what we think until the moment when the ideas of which they consist intervene effectively right in the middle of a session.

In contrast with those who do not write, there are those – here I am almost going to contradict myself – who imagine that writing consists simply in putting what one thinks down on a piece of paper. In any case, whether it's criticism, fiction or a psychoanalytic book, one never writes what one thinks but something else, because the construction of a text leads reflection in a direction that the author himself has not always foreseen. This does not mean that the initial project and the experience from which it arose were abandoned, lost en route, betrayed. On the contrary they may be seen, as it were, in perspective, and thereby gain in depth. And here we are brought back to the paradox of all writing: to attain this depth in the written text, in other words, to be a writer, whether psychoanalytic or not, it is certainly not enough to have ideas; but it is not enough either to be short of ideas.

P. – *You recognise, then, that the analyst can be engaged in writing which pursues, takes up again, assesses differently his activity of thought during the session. By doing this work, don't you have the feeling that you are necessarily distancing yourself from your mode of analytic functioning?*

M. – No, I don't think so. As you see, I am nuancing considerably my distinction between a literary text and an analytic text. Strangely enough, it is a negative phenomenon that makes it possible to compare the two genres: the psychoanalyst becomes a writer to some extent when he is inhibited in the course of his work. I am not speaking, of course, of laborious writing that is merely hindered by clumsiness. What I have in mind is those nagging blockages which suddenly call the whole person into question, disappear again soon after, just as suddenly, when one thought they had established themselves forever, and then reappear again not long after. Why all this torment if it is quite simply a matter of writing down one's reflections as they come to mind? If it was merely a question of accumulating pages, what obstacle could stop us on such a clear path?

P. – *But any such activity of "filling" deserves to be regarded with the same suspicion, whether it is filling pages or cramming one's daily schedule. Here, it is the compulsion that is a mark of the symptom; it is not the activity in itself. . . .*

The desire to write, for me, does not correspond to an overflowing of ideas that I have to get down onto the pages. It is more the opposite: a certain emptiness of thought or an excess of non-meaning. I do not write when "I am enchanted" but only when I feel disenchanted. . . . And this is closely bound up with practice. There can be a variety of general reasons such as uncertainty concerning the action we are taking; disappointment about the results obtained; the need to recover a personal sense of identity that has been put to the test and shaken, etc., but there are also some more particular ones. Certain phases of analysis, and sometimes even certain patients, stimulate the desire to write or even compel one to do so. But, paradoxically, it is not the most "stimulating" patients in sessions – those that facilitate associations, elaboration and interpretation in the analyst – that prompt us to write. It is wrong of me to say "paradoxically". In effect, when everything is played out on the analytic stage, why would one go in search of another? But when the stage of the session is no longer being used, when it is a desert or lacking in consistency, when the situation is too heavy, one feels – I feel – the need to get out of it, to get out of it without necessarily leaving it, as another activity would allow one to do. In my view, it is those patients who put us in difficulty who make us feel the need to write. It is a problem of countertransference, if you like; and also, if you will, an acceptable form of "acting out". But it may be that the recourse to writing has a comparable function to the recourse to the "supervisor" during the period of "training": speaking to a third party sometimes helps us to see what, without our realizing it, guides or limits our listening and our mode of intervention.

And then, taking up one's pen does not necessarily result in writing a text. Sometimes, just a "squiggle" or a few words put down on paper are enough.

But I have something else in mind: the work of writing. I understand it in the sense of the dream-work. When the analyst is writing, he must – and this does not happen without difficulty – carry out the very complicated operations that the dream accomplishes, as it were, spontaneously. For me, what is involved here is not at all a secondary, "literary" (in the weak sense of the word) elaboration that would add a small "aesthetic" touch to the product. That is why, although I am just as unconvinced as you are by certain attempts nowadays at analytic writing, I see in them a quest that interests me. I am not convinced because they are affected, deliberately sophisticated, and because "true" style is not something one chooses; it is the unconscious aspect of the text. But I am interested because analysts are finally tackling a problem that concerns them and whose solution cannot be delegated to professional writers. This problem is: how do we communicate the psychoanalytic object?

M. – We have been talking about what we transmit to others and also about what we may evoke in their minds; and also about the egotistical function of writing. Writing gives fresh impetus to our reflections, mobilises something in our practice and our thought in general, and also plays a part in our efforts at self-analysis. Is it sufficient to justify the undertaking itself and to induce one to continue it, for, in this respect, there is nothing like a second or third personal analysis? In any case, we cannot interest ourselves in the case of the analyst "who writes" ("*écrivant*") without evoking his narcissistic problems. And heaven only knows how sensitive the narcissism of analysts is: at least as much, if not more, than that of the writer. Writers and psychoanalysts are also exhibitionists and vain. They not only want to be recognised by others, but also to subjugate them. The analyst expects his writings to provide him with the narcissistic food of which he has a great need. And it is not impossible that the ups and downs of his practice increase his appetite in this respect. But by responding to this expectation, the others tend to lose their value as subjects, with the result that their praises very quickly lose their value and the author's narcissism is soon laid bare. Analysts readily acknowledge these considerations, and are even ironical and somewhat complacent about them. But I do not think that the wish to be published in order to be admired really throws any light on the need to write. It's a side issue. And the narcissistic situation is situated at an infinitely more serious level where, once again, the distinction between the analyst and the writer can be found. I was speaking earlier about the inhibitions that occur when one is writing and call the person as a whole into question. I am inclined to think that, in an individual who is in this situation, the blockages, the moments of rupture, are the reflection, as it were, of the breaches that are secretly tearing apart his narcissistic integrity. Bringing the work to its conclusion in spite of everything might very well have a sort of reparative virtue. We may ask ourselves if, in order to write, to really write, the analyst has to be ill? This may indeed be the case, but to a lesser degree, surely, than the writer. He never withdraws his interest in the world as much as the latter can do – the peculiar process of his writing does not require it, not to mention the fact that his patients do not allow him to do so. And if he sometimes identifies with his productions, he does not confuse himself with them or with their fate; it is as if effective safeguards, coming from one doesn't know where, opposed from a certain moment the progression of this movement. Writers, we know, or at least some of them, go a long way along this path. They sometimes regress deliberately, in their solitude, to the point of becoming fleetingly almost strangers to themselves. The analyst, for his part, writes during the day, and regresses primarily on another stage, when he listens to and accompanies his patients. Insofar as his frontiers are less threatened than the writers', and he is affected more deeply by the experience of depersonalisation,* the analyst does not have to treat writing as an absolute commandment.

Let me add one final word: and what if the analyst also writes because he has pleasure in doing so? After all, it's not forbidden!

. . .

Notes

1 Pontalis and de M'Uzan (1977) "Redirect, psychanalyser, écrire". When this interview first appeared in 1977 in the *Nouvelle Revue de Psychanalyse*, de M'Uzan, whose medical thesis in 1948 was on Kafka, had already published two works of fiction: *Les Chiens des rois* (*op. cit.*) and *Le Rire et la poussière* (*op. cit.*). In the year of the interview, he published, again with Gallimard, in the collection "Connaissance de l'Inconscient", *De l'art à la mort: itinéraire psychanalytique* (de M'Uzan, 1977).

2 Translator's note: In a short text titled "Ecrivains et écrivants", Barthes (1964) suggested that there are two forms of writer (and of writing) and created a distinction between the *écrivain* and the *écrivant*, that is, between the function of the author and the activity of the writer.

3 Translator's note: Arthur Adamov (1908–1970) was a playwright and one of the foremost exponents of the "Theatre of the Absurd".

4 Translator's note: An anonymous French novel written in 1678, often regarded as the beginning of the tradition of the psychological novel.

Chapter 2

The hell of creativity (2008c)[1]

The theme of "The artist and the psychoanalyst" – I would willingly say, psychoanalysis – began to interest me a long time ago, since my first contribution on the subject dates back to 1965 (de M'Uzan, 1965) and since then, in various circumstances, I have published the evolution of my ideas on this subject. And although I feel somewhat reticent about doing so, I must confess that my literary experience has contributed a great deal to my reflections.

The artist and his or her art is an immense domain in which one runs the risk of losing oneself, of putting forward propositions devoid of specificity or, at best, of "writing verse badly". Thus, without giving up possible digressions, I am going to circumscribe my theme closely. This theme is essentially related to what I consider to be the *nodal phase* of the activity in question, the primordial phase of what is called creative activity – I will come back to the expression, to the thing itself whose idealising aura leaves me, to say the least, with a number of reservations, which will not fail to come as a surprise. Not to mention the fact that although I am making an effort to understand the motive forces of creative activity, I want to emphasise that it will always escape our understanding. We will therefore pretend to believe in the legitimacy of the undertaking.

The *nodal phase* is related to phenomena in which the diverse artistic activities are rooted – artistic activities, and, no doubt, extreme scientific research. What, within the arts, distinguishes them from each other should depend on the development of their own history. That being so, I am led, while focusing mainly on the domain of writing, to adopt an "authoritarian" measure. This is a domain in which clearly I feel more at ease and which allows me, tactically, to delimit even further my theme – namely, *the rare poetic flashes at the heart of a piece of fictional writing*. The adoption of such a restrictive decision will no doubt invite criticism. In my view, it is indispensable if we want to try to understand, with a view to accounting for them, the specific phenomena, which, elsewhere too, will compel the person to bring into play original dispositions, including creative activity. And if I am narrowing the frontiers of creative activity to this extent, it is because, very soon, the artist, compelled to lie, to cheat and to pursue inadmissible aims, runs the risk of "tinkering with the incurable". From the beginning – and we will notice this again when we examine the process itself – the artist is first and foremost a victim, and the practice of art is the result of rigorous necessities; the artist has very little freedom and his or her destiny is fixed from the outset. Subsequently, the artist will certainly live through dramas that depend on various factors, dramas in which shame and guilt will weigh heavily.

But, to be brutal, the authentic artist, at least potentially, is the object of a malediction. In this respect the artist is comparable to the hero of Fritz Lang's (1931) film "*M*", who, faced with a jury full of crooks, screamed that he could not "do otherwise". It will be said, and not without reason, that I am exaggerating. This is inevitable if one wants to look at what is "elementary" or "initial", while thinking already of its extensions. I have even come to think that often the task of psychoanalysis is less to understand the causes of a failure than the lack of them when such a failure occurs. Consequently, everything becomes the object of a ruthless critical examination, and the reservations concerning the idealisation of creativity also concern for example the very mechanism of sublimation that underpins it. Freud (1923) had already noted this: "After sublimation, the erotic component no longer has the power to bind all the destructive elements that were combined with it, and these are released in the form of inclinations towards aggression and destruction" (p. 54).

Everything, therefore, has to be constantly taken up again. Joyce McDougall (2008) – who refers explicitly, it seems to me, to sublimation and applies it above all to the wish to possess both genders and to have children with both parents – notes the seriousness of the situation when she evokes the suffering of the artists that she had in analysis with her. But she takes an optimistic view of backing the powers of psychoanalysis to remedy it, since – and we will see this in examining the process – analysis is naturally in the service of the integration of the pregenital impulses in genitality. And since this operation is accomplished "ideally", it should, logically, deprive the artist of the "humus" in which the work of sublimation is anchored.

Having made these clarifications, I will move on to the creative process itself and to the primordial nodal phase that will set it in motion. The power, the empire of the phenomenon, is such that the totality of the person seems to identify with it, be reduced to it. The singularity of the matter, it will be understood, is, moreover, so extreme that one can only evoke it approximately, because the notions used to account for it belong to a vocabulary that is very familiar to us. The least uncertain is the term *depersonalization** – a-personalisation would even be more suitable, with its connotation of strangeness. The intimate, then, can no longer be distinguished from the extraterritorial; frontiers, limits and separations vanish, while immensity is reduced to a point. For a long time, I imagined that we were dealing with an issue linked to narcissistic drive functioning, that is to say, an issue that was still part of the psychosexual order. In the process I had noted the role of "seduction, most often by the maternal adult", as Jean Laplanche describes it; seduction that is at work during the emergence of the erogenous zones whose activity will require, and even compel, the psychic apparatus to invent the drive. Maternal seduction, which is excessively powerful or ambiguous, does not fail to confer on the said drive heavy pregenital characteristics, with little potential for evolution, which must imperatively be dealt with by the mechanism of sublimation . . . unless perversion comes into the picture! I cannot therefore follow Joyce McDougall when she says that it is the healthy part of the person that is creative. "Psychic health" is experienced in daily life, quite simply. One does not write as the bird sings! And in order to give you a feel for this, I will cite a few lines from two poems that come to mind in order to contrast them: one, depicting a perfect void, of which the author is José Maria de Heredia (1842–1905); the other, by Armen Lubin (1903–1974), whom I like to cite, and who does not have the honour of featuring in the *Petit Larousse*.

First, the extract from "The Trophies" (1900):

> And yonder, leaning against an arch under a bridge,
> Hannibal, thoughtful and triumphant,
> listened to the dull tread of the legions on the march.

And now, by Armen Lubin (1946), depicting audacious depth:

> When the lance bearers return
> Rainy Novembers,
> A learned dog, a huge dog
> Is making mysterious sums.
> He counts, he counts, he counts again,
> All sorrows are called absence
> All sorrows bearing lances.
>
> (translated for this edition)

Today, on rediscovering the initial intuitions whose theoretical implications could not at the time be fully recognised, while continuing to insist on the importance of what I have just been saying about the place and role of erotic drive functioning, I want to focus on what is *fundamental*, namely, the order of the *vital-identital*.* It is fundamental in more than one respect, but primarily inasmuch as it precedes, even if minimally, the sexual organisation, with which, in fact, its relations will be essential, albeit very complex. The order of the *identital*, it will have been understood, is to be distinguished from the narcissistic order which is part of the psychosexual register. It is thus related to the foundations of being, to the self-preservative sphere, I would say for the purposes of communication, and essentially involves a genetic programme that is promoted and guaranteed by the development of the soma, its protection and its preordained finiteness. This point is indispensable and is in keeping with an initial proposition of Freud to which he was to return in the first paragraph of Chapter 6 of *Beyond the Pleasure Principle* (Freud, 1920), where he places death on the side of the drives of self-preservation.

It is clear that the processes involved in "creative activity" do not develop within psychosexuality alone. The management of the pregenital partial drive impulses, through their sublimation, is undoubtedly an essential phase. But, in this matter, another process needs to be highlighted; namely – the term "drive"* should, in my view, be reserved for the psychosexual register – the process of what I have just called the non-instinctual drive *identital* that is extraneous to the narcissistic order, which implies a destiny and a placement of the libido. This *identital* concerns *being itself* to which we have access primarily at times when its shortcomings are in evidence, for example during phenomena of depersonalisation,* when everything vacillates, when a person loses his or her sense of their frontiers, leaving them connected with "psychic existence" only by the faculty of *perceiving* which is still intact. Within the fundamental sources of inspiration, or better, of an "authoritarian upheaval", there is thus a *disorder*. A disorder of identity, but also a phenomenon of an extremely serious economic nature that threatens even the creation of a double established previously in order to get beyond the primary state of confusion or lack of distinction (de M'Uzan, 1999) – I am speaking of the initial steps of the process and of what sets it in motion. What is involved is an indispensable rift or fault line that has not been healed or repaired and which continues to be a feature of one's being, in its very foundations, compelling the subject to represent him- or herself in order to survive. Traces of what is happening can sometimes be observed: an arrangement of screams, the irruption in consciousness of pictorial expressions in which one finally recognises a powerful entanglement of "border lines", or again, in front of the penholder, the imposition of a structure on the sentence, on the paragraph, awaiting contents to come that are eminently replaceable.

It is later that a story will have to be invented, imperatively, when the psychosexual, with its trail of perverse pregenital instinctual drive impulses, makes its pretensions known, by leaving, for example, sublimation with the task of dealing with the matter. Classical theses on creativity find their justification here. And we can find among them some of the views set out by Joyce McDougall, when she speaks of the decisive role played by the pregenital trends which, for her, are one of the four factors involved in any creative act – whether the empire of this universe, I would add, is linked to a fixation or proceeds from a temporal regression.

Regression: the word is out of the bag. Without libidinal regression, the so-called creativity is too much in danger of resembling an anti-cathexis or operational functioning (*l'opératoire*) (Marty & de M'Uzan, 1963), as I have been able to observe. A distant memory comes to mind here in passing: as a child, somewhat intrigued, I was watching the neighbour's small children, a brother and sister, who were carefully decorating the dog droppings in a cul de sac in Paris during the summer. They were planting "artistically" bits of matchsticks in them and placing tiny gravel stones on them in order to create sorts of small oeuvres. Were these the first steps of an active mechanism underlying a complicated work at the end of which one would find the smile of the "Mona Lisa"? Let me add that no provocation is intended here. But the evocation of this little scene once again gives me an opportunity to distinguish clearly between a child's creativity and that of the adult artist, whose filiation with this child is often asserted. The obvious complexity of the work of the artist who, nonetheless, is not at the heart of this study, has no counterpart in the child who, for his or her part, plays and looks towards the future, whereas the writer commemorates the past.* The pursuit of the construction of identity by the former stands in sharp contrast to the necessary dismemberment of identity in the latter – indeed this question deserves to be explored more fully.

To return to the creative process, as a whole and in its evolution, it can be argued that it is a product of the nature of the relations between a *drama of identity* and a *libidinal regression*, of the status of this "alliance", which like all alliances, is somewhat shadowy. Alliances, shared responsibilities: it does not require much thought to understand that the non-sexual drive disturbance of identity aggravates regression and affects the state of narcissism whereas, on the other hand, since regression is becoming more accentuated and love and hate are identifying with each other, the status of identity is altered. However fragile it may be, the effort to bring about a certain equilibrium in this relationship is vital; it is necessary, is it not, to escape as much from the abyss as from the demon? And the measures that the psychic apparatus has been led to adopt to achieve this are the very basis of creative engagement. Then comes, more familiarly, the rest of the adventure. I have recalled above the crucial place of pregenitality in this "adventure", the only aspect of sexuality to be sublimated.

An original psychic operation is carried out by the writer and is intended to create within a character, an inner figure, which is partly a product of parental images and of identification with cultural objects – and against which the writer can turn the most destructive impulses more or less with impunity. Sometimes we even see a fantasy emerging according to which the reader collapses on reading the first sentence, annihilated by its splendour. While the constitution of the inner character owes a great deal to the objects of the past, to the familiar cultural universe of the artist, it is nonetheless the equivalent of a *separate being*, distinct from the public itself. With this being, the artist will maintain specifically transferential relations, in the full sense of the term. These relations will be infinitely conflictual because, though, initially, the inner character, in its invention, was intended to participate in promoting the process – it will not be long before it transforms itself, at least in part, into the adversary of its creator; an adversary that the artist seeks to dominate or to whom he or she submits, and whom he or she even wants, tactically, potentially, to turn into an *alter ego* (it is here that references to unconscious homosexuality and bisexual fantasies have their place). A "fundamental complication" then appears when, as Murielle Gagnebin writes (Gagnebin, 2004, pp. 196–197, 278; 2011; Chantoiseau, 2014, pp. 19–36), the oeuvre in the course of "construction", and flourishing first of all as the *alter ego* of the artist, is "naturally led to transform itself into *Ego alter*", an *ego alter* that will dictate its desiderata to the artist, directing in part the work and imposing choices on her or him. Once again, it will be seen that creativity is far from being a happy undertaking.

I am led to consider the *pathology of creativity* – pleonastic? Let us nonetheless maintain the expression. It is heavy, admittedly, and yet, because it is paradoxically constitutive, it can turn out to be an impediment for the artist, the painter or the musician in exercising art; an impediment that exposes him or her, full of justifiable apprehension, to meeting the psychoanalyst. Joyce McDougall's observations are in this respect particularly demonstrative, albeit surprising theoretically since her patients who are "in an impasse" in the pursuit of their activity, as they are in their everyday lives, generally recover, thanks to analysis, their efficiency and even a certain happiness. This is perhaps an idyllic point of view, since certain "blockages" can, in effect, be removed thanks to analytic treatment. But, for the artist, who is more or less obscurely worried about the revolutionary foundations of the work, it may be better not to prolong the experience for too long. Georges Bataille said, did he not, to a certain writer who was exceptionally paralysed: "At last, the impasse!"? Alright, but, after all we should not forget that the deepest analysis does not go any further than the furrow of the labourer compared with the earth's crust.

Such considerations are no doubt somewhat disenchanted but, without returning to my comparison at a distance between José Maria de Heredia and Armen Lubin, it is my contention, once again, that the creativity of the child is almost entirely unrelated to that of the adult, which is not a "natural" creativity. Without dwelling on the "economic superiority" of the neurotic symptom – which has proved its worth over the long term – over the writing of a poem, it will perhaps be accepted, if we look at the contemporary world at least, that the behaviour of a large fringe of artists upholds the "power of disorder". Getting in touch with the primordial core of identity of a disturbing and frightening creative process, assuming the consequences of the indispensable libidinal regression, is no mean task: one has to work hard at it. And, as the undertaking has not been foreseen by nature, it is almost always necessary, in order to initiate it, to have recourse to artifice. That is to say, when it does not happen by itself, it is necessary to *provoke* the shaking up, the disturbance, of identity and its correlative libidinal regression by using chemistry. Absinth in the past – Freud thought for a while of using cocaine – today drugs, or a specific and intense form of physical exercise, or whatever. Publishers, gallery owners, have not thought as yet of introducing anti-doping controls. . . . But I am quite serious – there have been deaths by way of evidence – because a price will have to be paid (and soon also that of civilised means) for provoking (when it is necessary and using all available means, even the most dangerous) a fundamental disturbance affecting both the human being and the instinctual drives so that everything vacillates "usefully".

These last words could be conclusive. But if I limited myself to them, I would be exposing myself to the reproach of not having taken into account at all the role and the influence of the artist with the actual public that reads, and the public that visits galleries. My answer to such a reproach is that the relations in question are mediated, within a transference relationship with the "inner character" created, as we have seen, by the artist. We know very well that this public, over the course of the years, will make of the artist in succession, first a madman, then a prophet, then sometimes a pompous person, and finally a joker.

Note

1 This chapter was first published in French under the title of "L'enfer de la créativité" in *L'artiste et le psychanalyste*, Paris, Presses Universitaires de France (McDougall, 2008, pp. 35–46). It was republished in an adapted form in *L'inquiétude permanente* (de M'Uzan, 2015, pp. 34–42).

Chapter 3

Creative upheaval (2012)[1]

This phenomenon, over the course of the years, has often, directly or indirectly, held my attention, in respect of both its origin and its development; and yet I have never felt I have been able to identify its most extreme determinants. Literary writing imposed itself on me several years before I embarked upon analytic training and the analytic adventure. However, I am going to try again here to do so, while pointing out in advance that what I am going to say also concerns the other arts, and even science, in particular the "science of uncertain frontiers".

I shall only concern myself with one aspect of so-called creative psychic activity, namely, with the profound shaking up of being in its identity, with its "upheaval" (*saisissement*) and its strangely disquieting repercussions. I shall not therefore be dealing primarily, or even indirectly, with sexual drive processes or with sublimation, which I see as secondary phases, even though they are generally considered as the basis of the creative activity in question. The same is true of the notion of regression, which is so familiar inasmuch as it opens the path towards the part sexual drives, the only ones involved in sublimation.

This experience of upheaval refers to a moment, sometimes said to be "poetic", whether it is observed in the writer, especially at the heart of the prose from which it emerges and in which it is, as it were, lodged, or whether it is discovered, albeit more rarely, in the psychoanalyst, in the clinical work, but less in writings. It is the "degree zero" of the matter, as Roland Barthes (1953) put it.

In 1968, I recognised the phenomenon of creative upheaval as the corollary of a temporary libidinal regression, the consequence of the situation in the world of a being of desire. Today, while maintaining this point of view, I am looking further upstream – where the insistence of the subject is to be found – and I am concerned with the *nonsexual drive* essence of the experience of *creative upheaval*. Still more precisely, I am thinking of the relationship that links two "experiences": the second, the experience of uncanniness,* qualifying the first, the experience of creative upheaval, in order to give the subject access to another state of being; a human being, that is, who is involved in – has been precipitated into, I should say – an experience that leads him or her to the deepest and most serious aspects of him- or herself, while at the same time challenging the sensibility of those who are ready to leave the banks of the most concrete reality.

In trying to account for what happens in these circumstances, I am undertaking an exercise that is not "natural". A sort of unconsciousness, in the popular sense of the term, governs what I am evoking when one is not in control and when an imperious voice, coming from the most intimate depths of oneself, depths that are almost alien, dictates demands that I would describe as *formal*. They are formal to the extent that the content of the piece of writing counts less than its "architecture". The reader is invited here to see Murielle Gagnebin's reflections on the notion of *Ego alter* (see Gagnebin 2011).

What is the situation on the terrain of the experience itself? Take "Le Rire et la poussière" (in de M'Uzan, 1962, pp. 177ff.), a short story in which a specific link between laughter and obesity emerges. Incidentally, I imagine that this or that colleague will have divined some deep determining factor in this rapprochement; I can even imagine being capable of doing so myself by cheating a little with the abyss. Obesity, a theme that does not concern me personally in any way, except insofar as, one day, it organised my story, "Les Obèses du royaume" (ibid., pp. 91–138), having in mind the almost incomprehensible relationship between the enormity of bodily grease and a rare quality of expression. On the other hand, and resisting this profound ignorance, I knew, with the most severe assurance, that the beginning of the text in question would be long and consist of mutually engendering propositions, as if guided by a determining internal requirement ready to receive the contents to come.

One could speak of a *framework* offered for apparently random, albeit fundamentally imperious images which, subject to the requirements of a rhythm, burst into consciousness – a rhythm full of humour and possessing perhaps the meaning of the affair.

Thus, after having noted the evolution of the responsibilities distributed between the question of sexual drive activity and the question of identity, I was led to take into consideration fundamentally another relationship, that between upheaval and uncanniness. In itself, an upheaval is only potentially creative. As I have pointed out, it only acquires this power when it possesses, which is not always the case, a nameable evolutive capacity – the word is significant because, present within it, this potentiality is endowed with a natural appetite for words and verbs. An entity, in the full sense of the term, is thus built in which upheaval and uncanniness find themselves organically united. I call this experience the *crucial moment*; a crucial moment when the subject, emerging from the inexpressible, engenders this feeling of uncanniness in which creativity is ultimately rooted. Sublimation – which only concerns sexual drive functioning – is for later, or for elsewhere. Consequently, how can one fail to recognise the responsibility of a destiny? A destiny, first and foremost, that is linked or supported by the so-called quantitative factor, and when "I" is barely an "*every man's land*"[2] and not Winnicott's "no man's land".

Here are a few exemplary instants recalled by a woman analysand on returning from this experience. She said to me: "We are but one, owing to an effect of transparency. Each of us can be seen in the other. When each one is in the other, it makes but one". Less troubled, she continued, "It's funny, I lose my frontiers when I think about my relationship with you".

Another woman analysand said to me: "No, you are neither a friend nor an enemy, as could be the case in real life. . . . You are more an extension of me, you are part of me, yes, that's right. It's when you are part of me that I can imagine you, otherwise it doesn't work. After all, it's a way of being you". And on another day, she said: "No, you don't exist, except through me and in me".

In the midst of distressing disturbances of identity, another patient, as if devastated, managed to utter in a raspy voice the words: "I'm going to slip". Losing her contours, she was right in the middle of an experience of depersonalisation.* In the following session, ferocious hatred – albeit encouraging, if I may say so, for the object was beginning to emerge – was directed at the other, herself, and me, obviously. She was invaded by a powerful desire to destroy me, and I responded by saying: "You want to tear me apart within myself, where I in turn will cut you up into pieces". She was taken aback at first and then, in a whisper, she murmured a "yes", and I replied: "It's a question of appetite".

One day, an analysand cried out: "But what's happening today? I had the impression that I wasn't me". I replied: "You have probably lost me", and I heard him say: "Yes, no doubt . . . it's like those souls that change bodies or inhabit another. But would my thought no longer be in my body?" Another day, he let me know that he was only a part of himself.

In an utter state of dereliction, of total distress, a young woman murmured that "a hole had taken her place".

These words, and others besides, in no way owe what is essential in them to the pressure exerted – as I have already said – by an excessively strong and talkative sexual drive constitution. Although, in other situations, this may occur when obscure and significant narcissistic appetites have imposed themselves, which, having lost their libidinal quality, ended up inducing the *crucial moment*.

***

We discover several languages in a poem by Antonin Artaud titled "The Return of Artaud the Mômo" (1947), and that is why I often return to it. One of them, verging on a state of upheaval, consists of a series of onomatopoeia akin to a scream. Of the first of these languages I would say that it is an idiom of identity proffered by the "paraphrenic twin"* of the subject, succeeding the initial egotistical lallation – language that manifests, even if only fleetingly, the most authentic aspects of a person's being, lines that do not make one smile:

o dédi
a dada orzoura
o douzoura
a dada skizi
o kaya
o kaya ponoura
a pona
Poni

(Artaud, 1947, p. 13)

But there is another language, and in even more surprising forms, which already expresses the accession of the subject to the feeling of uncanniness. I will recall here part of what I had noted in "The Paraphrenic Twin" (1999) concerning the uncertain relationship between the world, the subject and his or her double.

Of that hoed bone that I am
In the filth
of a paradise
whose first dupe on earth
was not the father or the mother
who diddled you in this den
but
I
Screwed into my madness
And what seized hold of me
That I too rolled my life there
ME
NOTHING, nothing
Because I
I am there
I am there
And it is life
That rolls its obscene palm there
OK
And afterward
Afterward? Afterward?
The old Artaud
Is buried

In the chimney hole
That he owes to his cold gum
To the day when he was killed!
And afterward? Afterward?
Afterward!

(Artaud, 1947, pp. 18–19)

These lines call for silence. And yet, for other reasons, and after overcoming major reticences, I do not see how I can fail to allude, albeit very briefly, to another question whose significance is familiar to us all, to make an essential topic out of it. I am referring to the frequent, if not common, appetite for what is sometimes called "transcending oneself".

But does not transcending oneself – transcending oneself "in reverse" as it were – take us back to the sources of being, that "organic being" ("*das organische Wesen*", to use the term employed by Freud (1926) in *Inhibitions, Symptoms and Anxiety*) which is to be understood as the most fundamental aspect of the subject? It is as if the original fecundity – the fecundity, precisely, of organic being – was already in place first, or was acquired after a severe libidinal regression; in place, that is, at the *crucial moment* of which I have spoken. But things, far from it, do not always go like that. Since, for most people, this crucial moment is not naturally accessible or an inevitability, it is therefore necessary to induce it. And chemistry will cater for this: absinthe in the past, psychotropic substances today, and, I must insist, without the quality, or the part of the oeuvres thus induced, being affected in the slightest way.

Now that I have concluded the remarks I wanted to make or those that I have chosen to make, I must (defensively?) once again insist on the fact that I have only dealt with a part, admittedly fundamental in my view, of the questions engendered by so-called creative activities, some of which are called artistic. I have done so deliberately, with, as justification, the immensity of the subject, the conviction that I have identified what gravitated around the most essential aspects of it, namely, the creative upheaval, one of the psychic activities in which art, or the "artistic" is grounded.

Notes

1 This chapter was first published in *Michel de M'Uzan ou le saisissement créateur* (Gagnebin & Milly, 2012, pp. 15–20). It was republished in *L'inquiétude permanente* (de M'Uzan, 2015, pp. 43–49).
2 In italics in the original.

Chapter 4

The corrida . . . and its nether side (2011a)[1]

Barcelona, in that month of June 1962, hosted the 33rd Congress for French-speaking psychoanalysts. The city welcomed psychoanalysts who had escaped from other European cities to visit its beautiful austerity. And, to celebrate the event, the city also offered its guests the spectacle of a corrida.

Encouraged by my friends, and after overcoming a heavy feeling of hesitation, I accepted the invitation to discover something whose determinism I imagined to be complicated.

What I am about to say will, I know, offend – but that is inevitable – many of my colleagues, some of whom are friends; close friends, those of today, those of the past, *aficionados*, as we say. Consequently, I shall try to describe as coldly as possible what I saw unfold.

There was the arena, a very clear area covered with sand. There were multi-coloured stands surrounding it with rows rising up on all sides. There was the sky above, and it was a very beautiful day.

I am imagining a sense of expectation; I am imagining a silence. And then the memory forced itself upon me. In a blinding light, the gates of the bullpen opened wide, revealing a dark creature driven into the centre of the arena by its own momentum. The animal came to a standstill; it was the bull. With a nervous paw, the animal scratched the ground, raised its head, turned around, once, twice, lifted this head towards the sky to discover, finally, with its attentive gaze, an immensity that was still deserted. And the big animal had to wait, and wait again, perhaps without understanding, until a colourful entity came towards him. It was the torero, a man with a pronounced arch in his back, wearing a so-called "suit of lights" clinging tightly to his thighs and buttocks, embroidered with golden thread on his chest.

At the end of a short stick, a red cloth, a lure, taunted the animal which, perhaps, imagined a game; a game . . . until, a little later, the barbed sticks of the first banderillero were planted in its neck.

With his left foot forward, the man, moving sideways, escaped a first blind charge, followed by others from left and right, and still others that brushed the muleta closely with its humid nose. A dull scratching sound, seeming to come from distant times, rose from the stands, accompanying the ample and agitated movements of a bright red cape. It was a roar proffered by the crowd reduplicating the silences bound to time. The scenario was tightening.

The bull threw its powerful body against the caparison of the picador who was confined near the barriers in his own narrow space, lifted off the ground and about to be tipped over. The man, still mounted on his horse, aimed a barbed stick that was soon working its way into the shoulder of the animal, severing the ligaments of its shoulder.

The clocks were roaming chaotically, contaminated by the beating of hearts; they had seized power as if to manage the addition of the barbed sticks planted into and hanging from the body of a creature who, having lost the capacity to say no, was no longer quite the same.

The scene, imperceptibly, had shifted. A few steps away from each other, the man and the beast stood still. They faced each other, as if waiting for a new signal. And then, its pride perhaps lost, and added to its tiredness, the beautiful bull gave up fighting any more in an attempt to hold its head high, sufficiently, one more time. Finally, it lowered its head, offering its spine to what was going to be thrown at it: the long blade, still immobile, of the matador. A new silence imposed its law, briefly. And suddenly the absolute gesture unfurled, guiding an outstretched and plunging sword with the aim of planting it into the flesh. The big animal first collapsed onto its knees and then, as if being dragged along, its dark mass stretched out slowly, meeting the fate reserved for *it* since *the animal* came into the world. The sky was now reflected in its big open eye.

This is how, with deliberate solemnity, the story should come to a close. This is how a demanding ceremony should be accomplished. This is how a life has the task of witnessing for all lives. And, on this day, in this month of June 1962, in the austere city of Barcelona, an event was going to destroy the story by revealing a profound and unforeseen truth . . . and yet it was conveyed by a child who arrived and spat on the dark corpse, a mass of dead meat pulled outside the arena. A child spitting on the creature who, a short time before, had rushed into the light.

But it is absolutely necessary to return to the arena so that the story can be brought to a close, once and forever. In this month of June 1962, the matador, whose field of consciousness had no doubt been enlarged, revealed the hideous shadow of doubt that was invading him. He was extremely pale and his hand had become uncertain. But he was bound by a ritual that took over imperiously. What remained of him rushed, blindly, to thrust the sword into any part whatsoever of the bull's flesh. A jet of powerful blood began to pour out of the nostrils of the animal which, albeit completely wrecked, was still struggling. Then, from all the stands, the prolonged jeering of the crowd fell upon the man who, retreating, began to experience extreme humiliation, the humiliation of one who, without knowing it, was compelled to make us hear a message arising from the story.

It is with this message that I am henceforth concerned; a message that is sustained today by the image of a crowd pouring slowly out of the arena, like lava. Almost absent – I think I can imagine it – people are walking slowly, huddled together, like a huge creature, a dense substance, being led along nervously by guards on horseback. The image is harsh, and one would like to avert one's eyes from it. But memories impose themselves compellingly, just as sometimes in the psychoanalyst's consulting room, a thought or an image charged with undeniable density comes back to one's mind.

I am now back in 1934, in a town in Germany. July 1934, Hitler has become the new uncontested master of the country. In the towns, huge demonstrations are being organised, with their spectacular rigour. In spite of the accumulation of the passing years, the outline of the images is now becoming clearer. Dumbfounded, I recognise, in the brief and planned pauses of the speeches of yesteryear, the same deep roar, coming from bellies more than from throats, today scales the stalls of an arena and follows the rounded movements of a red piece of cloth.

Emden 1934, Barcelona 1962. The connection I am making with the demonstrations in this city is certainly intolerable. But when it is imposed by the drift of thoughts and a cruel memory, it means that the connection belongs to another order; an order situated at a more fundamental level than the unconscious, and yet ferocious. *"Au fond de l'homme, cela"*, Groddeck (1923) said, thinking of this unconscious, while the formulation concerned, first and foremost, a state of being; the "organic being", *"das organische Wesen"* of Freud who, without assured frontiers but armed with a biological blade, cut into it, and into his own flesh, before, being confronted with sex, with its emergence, he betrayed in order to be.

Note

1 This chapter was first published in French as an article in the *Revue française de psychanalyse*, 75, 1 (pp. 13–15) in 2011. It was republished in 2015 in *L'Inquiétude permanente*, pp. 57–64 (de M'Uzan, 2015a).

Part II

On the frontiers

Chapter 5

On the frontiers (2013a)[1]

Where am I? Who am I? Everywhere, nowhere. Once the line of questioning begins – defiance or insouciance – the state of blissful simplicity disappears . . . in favour of nowhere and everywhere. To call into question, seriously, the hypothetical notion of identity, something each one of us, without knowing it, believes he or she possesses, great frivolity or great madness is required, but this can come about. Let us imagine that it has occurred. Let us imagine it within our grasp, if I may put it like that, and the drama begins: "My frontiers are going to shreds". The woman who has come to see me in confidence encounters a rabbit's head lying in its blood, and in the process of dissolving in the pan. It is a part of herself:

> "It doesn't belong to me, and yet, it really is me", and she continues: "An unknown zone which is me but does not belong to me. It's as if, continuing to look at this part of myself, this part of myself was going to take precedence over the other, and then, that is all I would be". But who is this woman, where is she, this woman who, at other moments, is so wise, so reasonable?
>
> (de M'Uzan, 2015a, p. 57)

She *is* you, she *is* me, in search of herself, in search of her own identity, while making use of an antagonism with the not-self. This archaic self which has the task of differentiating itself from itself.

Was this not the case, right at the beginning, when it was necessary to extract oneself from *primordial being*?* Certainly, but at the beginning, at the very beginning, the task was fraught with risks.

That is the issue we will have to deal with when we are led to consider the impertinence of the question of the relations between *actual psychoses and somatosis*.

Pierre Marty, as we know, taking the order of mentalisation as his sole point of reference, shook up the existing nosography: "it's a matter of the heart *or* of the mind", he used to say. For my part, being less audacious, or more prudent, I imagine myself crushed between the outside, where I am not, and the inside, where I am too much. Would it not be better and wise, then, for a time, to be *nowhere*?

Furthermore, I think it would be useful to point out that "organised" psychoneuroses proceed from a "talkative" psychic functioning and, above all, that we are not dealing with several distinct entities, but with the manifestation of a true evolution according to which one passes over from primary anxiety hysteria, which is unstable and requires the implementation of psychic work, to phobia, a phobia that is the first stage of an *obsessional organisation*.

Between psychosis and somatosis (in the plural potentially), we are dealing with an immense territory in which – it is as well to remind ourselves – the symptomatology depends, partly, on the importance of the genetic factor. Are we then condemned to helplessness? No, for it sometimes happens that the prematurity of the human infant brings history into play – sometimes powerfully – a history that can make things swing one way or the other.

***

The theatre director, Bob Wilson, gave an interview about "Einstein on the Beach" (1976), in which he recalls his meeting with the musician Philip Glass.

In this interview, and it is almost caricatural, we can observe the *operational (opératoire) management* of the style, the enumeration of numbers, of time spans, everything being done on a note of quiet self-evidence with an extraordinarily impassive facial expression. Bob Wilson seems to introduce a sort of "operational defence", eventually directed against a psychotic swamping, a defence that then becomes the reason for his creation. Everything seems to obey a "mathematical logic", with "knee plays", as he calls them, which join two elements together. We are definitely dealing with a "combinatory system". It has been noted that he introduced *very detailed time spans*, which might suggest that Bob Wilson, ever *imperturbable*, may have experienced a necessity of an *operational order*, that is to say, referring only to the most concrete aspects of reality. Three references to trains seem to bear this out; but it is as though he had no choice. Certainly, trains are an ordinary means of transport, but we know the polysemy of the word transport; just think of erotic forms of transportation! So are we dealing with the danger of psychotic swamping or of an operational defence? Bob Wilson soon shatters the image of the train by speaking of the structure of a building. It then becomes a matter of the symbolic meeting, but how difficult that is, of two objects, of two beings! What is of fundamental interest is the *descriptive coldness* that affects Bob

Wilson's statements, attesting to a hypercathexis of the factual that is characteristic of the operational subject.

***

In order to explore these themes in greater depth, I want to study the second part of an important work by Bob Wilson called "Deafman Glance", created in 1970 in New York and in Paris and shown on television in 1981.

The theme of "Deafman Glance" is as follows: a woman (a mother? a nurse?) offers a child a glass of milk twice. We see her pouring the milk with great care into each glass. We hear very loudly each noise coming from the kitchen: dishes, putting plates away, opening the fridge, lighting the gas, as well as the sound of her footsteps on the stairs leading to the bedrooms and that of the rustling of the material of her baggy dark dress. These noises are amplified, while at the beginning and ending of the film, we hear normal noises from *outside* (birds or crickets singing). Having brought the glasses of milk, the woman then equally mechanically puts a knife through the child who is either sitting on a chair reading a book or sleeping on a bed.

What is this work about? The slowness, the icy presentation of the images and of their sequences leaves the spectator thoughtful and perplexed as to their purpose.

For some – it has been said – it is a feminist caricature of the place of the woman in American society. A number of theoreticians have used this caricature to argue that the filmmakers of this era chose to film a woman's work in almost real time (peeling a potato, preparing a bath, etc.). But there is *a quite different point of view* according to which we are dealing with the implementation of a programme in which the "sexual", strictly speaking – in Jean Laplanche's[2] sense – seems to be *completely absent*: the knife, filmed close up, would be like an anti-body. It seems to penetrate a foreign organism without, however, producing a haemorrhage. At any rate, what we think about is the *execution of the work* and the *contrasts* it contains: first the slowness, which is pronounced and thus full of meaning. The role of the amplification of noises, frozen frames of objects such as the glass of milk filled to the rim, the knife painstakingly washed, the work of the camera alternating between general views and high angle close-ups. Nothing is left to chance, everything is carefully controlled, right down to the nuances of grey and white. A light bulb, at the end of its wire first hangs immobile before our eyes and then, suddenly, this wire bends strangely as if propelled by a powerful extradiegetic blast of air – a moment in which it is legitimate to conceive of the place of the psychosexual. Likewise, there is an intense noise of gas leaking from the gas cooker, revealed by a high angle and very close-up shot. We can also note the contrast between the chirping of the birds off-camera during the initial film credits and those of the crickets at the very end. There is thus a different way of treating the natural noises, outside the house, and the amplified noises coming from the woman who goes up and down the stairs. Once again, are we faced with the projection of the inner world of this woman (a mother?) or with her powerfully controlled delusion? Think of the creaking of the parquet, of the noises of shoes on the floor, of the rustling of the material of which the long dress with large shoulder pads is made. We may also mention the various noises of the clattering of dishes, of water leaking from the tap, of the tea towel thrown onto a pile of plates and of the motor of the fridge when its door opens – a door that would only close again later on and strangely all by itself with a strong creaking noise. Extradiegetic music intervenes when the child, who is sitting, begins to turn the pages of the album resting on his knees, while the woman hands him a glass of milk and placidly bumps him off (first part of the film). The music intervenes a second time when the woman is preparing to plunge once again a knife into the body of the child who at this point is lying on his bed (second part of the film).

In the second part, the extradiegetic cello begins when the child, sleeping in his bed, is awakened by the woman who hands him a glass of milk which he takes. The cello starts again at the point when the woman with the knife enters the bedroom of the child, who is lying down, with the aim of murdering him.

Let me repeat, the different contrasts of sounds (natural noises outside the house, birds chirping, crickets singing; diegetic noises in the house, all highly exaggerated; and finally the emergence on four occasions of a few bars of cello, always extradiegetic) appear violently and play a large part in the strangeness of the performance.

There is also the moment when the woman carefully wipes the blade of the knife until it reflects her face. We are therefore justified in asking ourselves if the confrontation with the specular image can be interpreted as representing the meeting with the double – the murder of two children, it is plausible – a double announcing the emergence of the *paraphrenic twin*.* This notion defines a psychic being whose traces persist throughout the history of an individual. These traces are less evident than those of the pregenital phases of libidinal development, but clearly identifiable when the figure of the double suddenly emerges (de M'Uzan, 1999).

We may wonder why Bob Wilson's extremely elaborate aesthetics leave some spectators cold and distant. If that is the case, a *larger* place, perhaps, should be reserved for the entity that I have called *actual psychosis*,* that is to say, an actual psychosis that is not strictly speaking explicitly delusional and has its place between the somatoses and the delusional psychoses or alongside them.

***

Another film, this time by the film director, Martin Scorsese, "*The Big Shave*" (1967), allows me to reflect on what is often a daily activity for men. Against a background of light and relatively catchy jazz music from 1937 by Bunny Berigan ("I Can't Get Started"), we discover the décor of a bathroom. In succession we get a view of the W.C., a shower tray, a towel rack, a roll of toilet paper, the shower head, taps and finally a mirror. A man, a quiet man, is approaching the mirror in order to have a shave. A banal activity, if ever there was one, and yet ideas of hygiene, of narcissistic, or even seductive, exigency are initially involved – and in what an order! – which implies the role of the *sexual*. Until the end, it is as if, for the man, there was no absolutely no doubt about the banality of the activity. And yet, with this film, nothing could be further from the truth.

The activity begins in the most ordinary way. There is a first, slight cut. Nothing but very ordinary. Then as the activity continues, the scene changes: he cuts himself more and more badly. His face becomes a wound, but the man remains impassive and the sink fills up with blood – a reference, albeit in another register, to Hitchcock's 1960 film "*Psycho*". The scene ends at the moment when, with blood stains even on his feet and blood running down his chest, the man calmly puts the razor down on the edge of the sink. Both these scenes are shown in two very big close-up shots sectioning, once again, the man's body, as if place prevailed over being.

Faced with these scenes, each man (each woman, why not?) may feel, let's say, dumbfounded. And consequently, and no doubt with the aim of wresting back the advantage, an effort of theorisation is necessary – a defence, as it were. With the initial scratch, we may suppose that the place of the *sexual* has to be taken into account, which is reassuring.[3] Soon, and *progressively*, the adventure evolves for, from the possible reference to castration, we move forcefully and rapidly on to a destructiveness that is highlighted in a remarkable way by the man's impassibility. The haemorrhage, the increasing amount of dripping blood, is *substituted* for the man who is summed up, expressed by his blood. And I am not far from thinking that the man in question might be nothing more than the plughole of a sink. A hitherside of the inert that only horror, a virtue, could contain.

We can find a striking expression of this horror in the first pages of *Kotik Letaev* by Andrei Biely, who evokes the ineffable appearance of the life of the newborn baby in these terms:

> The first "*thou-art*" grips me in imageless deliria; and – in age old immemorially familiar ones: inexpressibilities, unprecedentednesses of consciousness lying in the body, the mathematically exact sensation that you are both you and not you, but . . . a kind of swelling into nowhere and nothing, which all the same is not to be mastered, and – "What is this?".
>
> (Biely, 1915, p. 9)

Let us take a final example to back up my remarks. "Fase", a choreography (58 minutes) by Anne Teresa de Keersmaeker – a major piece in the history of contemporary dance (160 productions since 1982) – was set to Steve Reich's early music work. A video was created by Thierry De Mey in 2002.

Two dancers, whose silhouettes are multiplied by lighting effects, evolve into repetitive and strictly controlled figures. This work revolves around a duo executing simple movements – walking, twisting, swaying of arms – and is also organised according to elementary geometric constructions (tireless repetitions of a few motifs). The dancers are Anne Teresa de Keersmaeker and the videographer's sister, Michèle De Mey.

In this filmed extract, the movements sometimes verge on a loss of balance. The extreme formalism of the gestures, their repetitive rhythm, create a hypnotic state in the spectator that sometimes borders on boredom; but only sometimes because we may be led to wonder if we are not on the path of a repetition which, ultimately, will result in opening out on to the *same*.* Such repetition often involves *small* variations, *small* alterations recognising depth of field (blue shadow among others, as well as their multiplications). We may see in this the beginnings of an opening on to the "sexual" (impediments controlled by the music, imperceptible movements of dresses, height of socks, variations of tennis shoes filmed in close-up, agitation of the hair of the two women, etc.). The presence of the other can be identified: the two silhouettes project shadows which are multiplied and superimposed. Is it legitimate to imagine a meeting between two characters, or alternatively, another hypothesis, to conceive of the emergence of being itself through a manifestation of the paraphrenic twin?* The "paraphrenic twin" results, in my view, let me recall, from a complex psychic operation through which "the archaic self will be able to emerge from primordial being and forge the beginnings of a distinctive identity" (de M'Uzan, 1999, p. 105).

But the sphere of the *vital-identital** prevails: these works do not aim to recount anything or to go anywhere. We are thus confronted with a simple mode of functioning that persists.

Notes

1 This chapter was first published as an article in the *Revue française de psychosomatique*, 43, pp. 23–31, in 2013.
2 See Laplanche (2007). The word "sexual" used by this author refers to everything that belongs to the extended Freudian theory of sexuality. It thus designates the primacy, in psychoanalysis, of a unique and specific variety of sexuality which is at the heart of the notions of the drive and of the unconscious.
3 But what a contrast with the scene in John Huston's 1951 film *The African Queen*, in which Humphrey Bogart is shaving happily while thinking about Rose, interpreted by Katharine Hepburn!

Chapter 6

A new perspective in psychoanalysis (2008b)[1]

Having reached a certain age, and with the benefit of long experience, one can see how, over the course of the years, ideas have imposed themselves, leading on to others, without always having been anticipated. This being so, we would be justified in pleading not guilty. In any case, these ideas were sufficiently insistent to make one pay close attention to them. And this is why I have not been able, for example, to avoid noting certain incoherent elements in the analytical corpus, as it has been handed down to us. Hence the title of this chapter.

Major imprecisions and contradictions can, in fact, be identified, not only within the two topographies and the two theories of the "instincts", but also, and above all, between the two stages of the Freudian edifice. It was therefore inevitable that one day a concern for consistency would arise, even if, for a long time, for far too long, we had adjusted to the situation. This concern for coherence gave rise to a compelling need to elaborate, at the risk of an excess of audacity, a sufficiently ordered "theoretical edifice". Let me explain myself. Consider, for example, the situation concerning the famous *death drive.** Is it not striking to notice that Freud (1920), in *Beyond the Pleasure Principle* (Chapter 6, first paragraph), places death on the side of self-preservation, only to renounce this hypothesis immediately afterwards by positing a second theory of the drives of which he says (all within the same chapter) he is not sure he believes himself? Perhaps, and even more serious, if I may say so, is the blow inflicted by the second structural theory of the psychic apparatus (ego, id, superego) on the discovery of one of the most fabulous findings in the history of thought: the recognition of the Unconscious, of the systemic Unconscious, with all its distinctive elements (absence of the notion of past, non-representation of death, etc.). As we know, it was a discovery whose importance equalled that of the two other narcissistic wounds inflicted on humanity, first by Copernicus, then by Darwin (see Freud, 1917). This discovery was poorly tolerated, even by analysts, as evidenced by the employment of this notion of systemic Unconscious in the second topography where the Unconscious – without ceasing to exist? – becomes a *quality* that can be recognised as much in the ego as in the superego and the id. Such an evolution provides food for thought, and it is an opportunity to recall with Ernest Jones that, if Freud had died just after writing the great metapsychological papers of 1915, we would have possessed a complete picture of psychoanalysis in its classical form. Thus, when a theory has proved its worth, the discoveries that come after it cannot substitute themselves, or even simply be added, to the first edifice. It is necessary, then, before retaining them, to evaluate how far they can be integrated "organically" with the first theoretical construction. Psychosomatic medicine is a good illustration of this and can even serve as a call to order. Psychoanalysts, who are very much at ease with the topographical and dynamic points of view, are much more embarrassed by the economic point of view, that is, by the fact that quantity can be a mark of destiny; though quantity, it will be said, is more easily induced than measured. Psychoanalytic psychosomatic medicine, it is true, manifests a unifying purpose by grouping together as part of the same order the somatoses, the psychoneuroses and even the psychoses. Such an approach should help to avoid falling into the error of placing this or that patient into a nosographical category to which he or she does not belong.

By way of example, I would like to evoke two old and comparable anecdotes. Two mentors, who have since passed away, contacted me one day for the same reason. Both of them knew about my interest in psychosomatics. These two fine clinicians had diagnosed an obsessional neurosis in their respective patients, since all the semiological elements were present. At once intrigued and distressed, they had both observed the onset of a very serious bout of ulcerative haemorrhagic colitis in their patients, one of whom was nearing the end of his analysis, and the other in the middle of his analysis. What had happened? I could only suppose that a part of the economy of these patients had escaped their attention. Indeed, everything that belonged to the obsessional neurotic register had been worked on and analysed, but it had only required an event of an economic order (probably an intervention) to overwhelm the adaptive capacities of the obsessional system, which collapsed like a house of cards, for the whole economy to shift elsewhere. I could, as could others, evoke many similar situations. Such miscalculations call for reflection and underlie the notion of psychoanalytic psychosomatics, with its vocation of unifying two universes. Consequently, it took more than one day to reach the point at which a sufficiently coherent unifying theoretical conception could be established. This is by no means a recent quest because I have found traces of it dating back to 1969 in a paper I gave at a colloquium of the Paris Psychoanalytical Society devoted to the *compulsion to repeat*. The links between this notion and the death drive* seemed self-evident. I remained puzzled, hesitating to follow the movement, first because my clinical practice presented me regularly with phenomena of repetition whose understanding did not in any way require recourse to the role of a particular drive (the so-called death drive); and secondly, because I preferred to refer to the clinically identifiable opposition between phenomena of "repetition of the identical"* and those where the repetition is approximative – the same* (see *same* and *identical* in the glossary) – an opposition that can be found in the dictionary. So I left the question of the death drive for other occasions, thereby exercising caution – elementary caution, in fact, which makes it possible in later writings not to remain a prisoner of the initial positions one has adopted. It was necessary, therefore, at the time, to allow space for critical reflection; in other words, to engage in some reflection and then to begin accumulating observations with a view to submitting them to close and attentive scrutiny. This was the case when, for several years, Pierre Marty, Christian David and myself analysed, week after week, the recordings of preliminary interviews with predictably "psychosomatic" patients in the neurosurgical department of Prof. Marcel David. Part of this work appears in *L'Investigation psychosomatique* (de M'Uzan, Marty, & David, 1963),[2] which has since become a classic. It was in these conditions that the operational mode of thinking (*pensée opératoire**) was detected and then analysed. A few years later, Dr Nemiah's team, from Harvard, who had been informed of our studies by Dr Mertens de Vilmar (Liège), reconsidered his own observations and recognised in turn the phenomenon of operational thinking.

I have identified several themes, the first of which is a reminder of the fundamental specificity of the "systemic Unconscious". To avoid any ambiguity, I will recall the two oppositions corresponding to the two major phases in Freud's thought. According to the first, self-preservation/psychosexuality accompanies the topographical distinction between unconscious, preconscious and conscious. According to the second, "life instinct/death instinct" accompanies the distinction between id, ego and superego. The two topographies and the two instinctual drive (*Triebe*) theories do not overlap at all. How can they be made to coexist? I believe, along with Francis Pasche, that ego, id and superego can be taken for characters involved in a scenario, whereas conscious, preconscious and unconscious are their modes of functioning, in other words, their *mise en scène*. Furthermore, one would have to accept, again with Pasche, the employment of the term "drive" (*pulsion*) *only* for "partial" drive engagement (epistemophilic drive, etc.), while the term "instinct" should be reserved for the life instinct and death instinct (see the "essentially genetic programme" below). To sum up – hygiene of thought – with all the contributions following the major metapsychological papers, it is necessary to evaluate whether, and to what extent, they can be integrated with the first topography without having a negative impact, in other words, with the complete theoretical edifice of which Jones speaks. An illustration, among many others, of the issue in question, concerns the admission of

Melanie Klein to the International Psychoanalytical Association. Edward Glover – whose book on technique deserves the closest attention – was opposed to it, and not without reasons. Ernest Jones, a great diplomat, succeeded – fortunately perhaps – in reversing the situation. Melanie Klein was accepted by the IPA. And yet her views – on child development, for example – were far removed from those that can be deduced from Freud's work. How, indeed, is the Kleinian idea of a *linear* development for the different stages passed through in perfect continuity from the pregenital stage to the phallic stage – where she speaks of an "early Oedipus complex" – to be reconciled with the Freudian perspective where the evolution occurs through mutations, the major mutation being that of the Oedipus complex itself, when the whole of the pregenital past is "destroyed" and rewritten in terms of threats of castration and castration anxiety (de M'Uzan, 1988)? What has been experienced in archaic reality is not accessible as such; indeed, what we are dealing with is a tendentious and misleading account of it. It is up to each analyst therefore to take up his or her own position, for interpretive activity as a whole will depend on it.

It is customary to translate the German word *Trieb* by *pulsion* in French. This initiative, taken by the linguistic commission of the Paris Psychoanalytical Society (SPP) in 1927, was the result in fact of hard negotiation: "If you give me *pulsion* for *Trieb*, I will accept *Ça* (in place of *soi* [self]) for *Es* (Id)". The matter is not without significance, since in German, *Trieb* is a popular term compared with the scientific word *Instinkt*, whereas in French the contrary is true. However, and in order to be rigorous, if "instinct" may at a pinch be suitable for life or for death, the use of the word *"drive"* (*pulsion*) must, on the contrary, in order to be legitimate, correspond to the metapsychological requirements described in "Instincts and Their Vicissitudes" (Freud, 1915) (source, aim, pressure, object).[3] *Drive* only concerns the object-related and narcissistic psychosexual order. It is thus logically unacceptable to speak of a "drive" of self-preservation and, all the more so, of a death drive.*

It is now time to propose a theoretical/doctrinal edifice that articulates the different notions evoked. This can be done in the form of a fable. At the moment when male and female gametes meet each other, an essentially genetic programme is set up to organise in advance the development and finiteness of being without any other drive-based intervention. Self-preservation, only, defines *one* of the responsibilities featuring in the programme. The energy involved in the adventure is, at the outset, *without quality*; in other words, it is put in the service of the functioning of the organism, brain included. Part of this energy *is waiting* to be "qualified", that is to say, it anticipates acquiring a libidinal status. On the trajectory of the programme, stages are, as it were, foreseen, as well as accidents (genetic illnesses, for example). One of the most important is the appearance of the erogenous zones. We can imagine the situation in terms of the model of the "cell" as a lock waiting for the "viral key". The lock, in the programme (which some would call self-preservative) is ready to become an actual erogenous zone thanks to the intervention of the seduction of the *infans* by the adult, most often the mother. The decisive role of this seduction has been studied and described at length by Jean Laplanche (1987). For him, the message addressed by the adult, during moments of infant care in particular, is contaminated by his/her unconscious, and leaves a remainder to be interpreted by the *infans*, on the basis of which the latter's unconscious will begin to establish itself.

While I recognise without any reservations the role of the seduction of the *infans* by the adult, as Jean Laplanche has described it and developed the issues involved in it, I am concerned primarily with the responsibility of this seduction in the appearance, sifting out and emergence of the erogenous zones in the genetic programme, where the occurrence of the phenomenon was foreseen. As a result, the quantity of the work that the activity of these erogenous zones imposes on the psychical apparatus will transform the energy "without quality" into what we call the *drive*, a drive that is always sexual. As we know, Freud defined the drive economically as the "demand made upon the mind for work in consequence of its connection with the body" (1915, p. 122). In so doing, energy, without quality to begin with, becomes libidinal drive energy, animating the essential aspects of what is played out in the psychosexual order, while its locus of cathexis will identify it either as object related or narcissistic. Concretely, in everyday practice, we are primarily dealing with clinical pictures in which we can discern interactions, "negotiations"* between energies – without quality – of functioning and sexual libidinal drive energies. Thus, in the psychosomatic domain there are organs that are almost silent, the kidneys for example, while others, endowed with language, can be psychosexually very talkative, such as the so-called "irritable" colon. Finally, and to make things even clearer, there are grounds for positing that the drive is an *invention* of the psychical apparatus which, as Freud claimed, is a *fiction*.

This, then, is the theoretical framework – the fable. Among the important subjects that must find their metapsychological place within this framework, some have already been discussed, but it is necessary to return to them. The first is "operational" thinking (*pensée opératoire*) in that, on the face of it, its characteristics are not such that we can recognise its place in the psychosexual order, while a strictly metapsychological view of the phenomenon suggests something quite different. Next comes what I shall call the "problematic of identity". In connection with this subject, I will make a few brief remarks on non-delusional psychoses; finally, I will recall certain distinctions in the psychic work that those who are approaching death are sometimes led to undertake.

Although operational thinking is alien to psychosexual functioning and although, in spite of this fact, we return metapsychologically to the fundamental characteristic of the operational phenomenon, that is to say, the hypercathexis of the most factual aspects of reality, there is reason to suppose that the perception of reality must have been threatened by, and exposed to, an extreme danger, namely, the emergence of a hallucination. Only an archaic mechanism possesses such power. The mechanism in question is the Freudian "*Verwerfung*" (which Lacan interprets with the concept of "foreclosure"), the "*Verwerfung*" or rejection of an ideational content or signifier that may reappear hallucinatorily. Operational thinking is thus a defence against the consequences of a psychotic defence (see de M'Uzan, 1974b).

Just as, with operational thinking, interpreted metapsychologically, I had integrated organically the somatic and psychosexual orders, I would like to reconsider the subject's "problematic of identity". This requires me to draw attention to a confusion whereby we speak of narcissism, linked to the fate of the libido, instead of this dimension of identity which concerns what I call the "*vital-identital*"* (or the self-preservative field). In *Inhibitions, Symptoms and Anxiety* (1926), Freud speaks of "organic being". Disregarding this distinction can lead us astray when it is a matter of the frontiers between the respective domains and of the natural uncertainty that affects them. Here is an illustration.

When, having got off the couch at the end of her session, a seriously depersonalised woman patient managed to describe the emotions that were overwhelming her, I said to her "simply": "Your contours are in my pocket", choosing to direct my intervention towards the frontiers of her being and the fact that they were not lost. Experiences of uncanniness express best those moments in which the *vital-identital* and the psychosexual are both involved, with indefinite frontiers. This grants psychoanalysis, alongside biology and even mathematics, the right to belong to the "scientific domain of indefinite frontiers" (see de M'Uzan, 2009). The random character, albeit difficult to identify, of the frontiers generally considered as well established is understandable when an extremely serious complication occurs affecting the transplant of haematopoietic stem cells (HSCT), indicated sometimes in cases of child leukaemia (see Ascher & Jouet, 2004). Contrary to the most frequent complication, it is no longer the subject who rejects the transplant, but the transplant, having become subject, that rejects the subject who has become the other, the stranger, with a fatal outcome in which the child is "skinned alive".

If I am allowing myself now to take a brief look at the non-delusional psychoses, it is because consideration of the nosographical point of view, based on the particularities of psychic functioning, justifies once again the wish to include within a single framework neurotic, psychotic and psychosomatic pathologies as a whole. The reader will find an exposition of these views in de M'Uzan (2005a). Thus in opposition to the classical contrast between actual neuroses and psychoneuroses, I would set actual psychoses/paraphrenias and imaginative delusions. In both cases, the significant contrast proceeds from the psychic work involved. Either it is of an "operational" nature and the symptom has no significant value, or it is fully mentalised and the symptom is sufficiently eloquent to describe a scenario. The reader will have recognised, more or less, in what I have called "actual neuroses",* the "cold psychoses" described by Evelyne Kestemberg (2001).

The reader will perhaps be surprised to see me close my remarks by broaching the theme of death or, more precisely, the work of dying.* It is no secret that I have already dwelt on this topic on several occasions (de M'Uzan, 1968, 1976a, 1981, 1996). I hope that this will not be seen as a choice of preference. It was a matter of chance, and my first publications on the subject undoubtedly led me to consult a number of people who had been informed of their inescapable and forthcoming demise. The issue, for several of them, was clearly to initiate a final "work" – the word is out, and that is exactly what is involved – on themselves. But more than that was necessary to support my decision to return to the subject in this chapter; I am referring to a cardinal theme in everything that I have just been saying, namely, the nature of the work in question, the state of the problematic of identity and the place of seduction.

To put things rather abruptly, among the persons who came to see me in this tragic context, there were those who "did not want to die" and those who "wanted to go on living" – living psychically, that is, by making use of all the instruments of phantasmatic functioning, of mentalisation, that was still available to them. In fact, as things unfolded, both modalities were present, but with a clear predominance of one or the other, *right up until the end*. There is therefore no reason to be surprised if "those who do not want to die" develop primarily an "operational" type of psychic functioning, whereas those whose capacity to fantasise, to dream, is better preserved, pay for it neurotically. Is it not rather astounding that a certain patient, who had been informed that she would die shortly, expressed clearly and unambiguously the wish to get to grips with neurotic symptoms that had only partly been resolved during an earlier analysis (de M'Uzan, 1981)? Another patient, a few hours before his death, was wondering with me about the meaning of a "memory image" of a shoe with a silver buckle.

What I am about to say may seem shocking, due to the sense of unease caused by referring to seduction within analysis itself. Nonetheless, I must deal with the issue. It is worth noting to begin with that the mere fact of addressing oneself to another person, in whatever context (or almost) inevitably comprises an element of seduction, and I do not need to remind you of the decisive role of seduction in the first stages, already, of the life of the *infans*; a role that is not lost over the course of the years. This can be sometimes be seen in extreme situations such as those to which I have just referred: the approach of death. As evidence of this I will take the case of a woman invaded by metastases who, generally speaking, had little interest in the work of mentalisation, but who was now quite attentive to what might keep one in ignorance of a fatal outcome. And yet, at certain moments, just as openings may suddenly appear in a cloudy sky, she let herself express something seductive in a fantasy life that was otherwise too restricted. So I decided to take advantage of this situation by accepting, after validating her narcissistically, a certain degree of eroticisation in the exchange. Unfortunately, I have to admit that this time the initiative, underpinned by an authentic engagement on my part, failed, at least in part: soon enough, hard reality, in all its aridity, would orient the medical approach towards a decision to gradually "put her to sleep".

I would like to conclude these lines by evoking a personal memory, an old memory, foreign to the psychoanalytic world, but one that often comes back to me. It is the memory of a young woman, a friend who passed away after succumbing to metastatic breast cancer. She was a journalist and novelist from an Eastern European country who had closely escaped a fate that it is not difficult to imagine. I will leave to one side my role in the discovery and treatment of the first tumour in order to concentrate on what specifically concerns my subject. Even though the illness was already in a very advanced state of progression and my friend was unaware of its impending fatal outcome, she made the acquaintance of a surgeon who had no connections with the medical and surgical team that was taking care of her. Curiously enough, I was able to recall this surgeon's thesis ("Non-tuberculous Purulent Pleurisy"), which I had read and admired during my medical studies, having been impressed by the intelligence and sensibility that it revealed. And it was he, strangely enough, who was to inform my friend of the seriousness of her state and of its imminent outcome. Even more strangely, and to everyone's surprise, a genuinely loving relationship, emotional and sexual, developed between them. Intrigued at first, I soon understood that the man, who was sensitive to the powerful charm of the young woman and genuinely smitten, had understood with extraordinary intuition that it was within his power to "leave the paths of reason" by transforming the organic drama into a situation in which the psychosexual conserved its place infinitely.

The young woman was to give an ultimate illustration of all this richness. A few days before her death, her last book had just been published, but still wanting to ensure its promotion, she had herself taken by ambulance to her publisher's. One of the doctors in the department where she was hospitalised accompanied her with two nurses, all of them trembling at the thought of what might happen. And in one of the salons turned into a studio, under the spotlights, and in the midst of all the journalists, my friend, radiant, elegantly dressed, brilliant and still seductive, could be seen subjugating everyone in attendance.

Notes

1 This chapter first appeared in 2008 as a paper in the *Bulletin du groupe méditerranéen de la Société Psychanalytique de Paris*, 17, pp. 9–17. It was republished in *L'inquiétude permanente*, 2015, pp. 65–76.
2 The second and third editions from 1994 and 2015 include an additional text by David and de M'Uzan titled "Préliminaires critiques à la recherche psychosomatique".
3 Translator's note: In French, *Pulsions et destin de pulsions*.

Chapter 7

Introduction to the theory of the preliminary interview (2010)[1]

The man arrives. I know nothing about him. I do not want to know anything about him.

It is not always like that. I regret it. But what can I do?

But where does he come from, this man who has come to see me, who me? Who of me?[2] What does he want from me, this man, as if it were a drama or an adventure? If I forget him, nothing will be illuminated and, like an ant, I will scratch the soil indefinitely; forgetting will come. I will not know any longer that we form only one single merged being, as close as possible to what we are, when we were.

***

The considerations that I am going to present on the preliminary interview for a psychoanalytic treatment are the result of very long experience (more than sixty years) acquired mainly in private practice, but also in so-called "hospital" settings: at the Jean Favreau Centre for Consultations of the Paris Institute of Psychoanalysis; at the centre for psychoanalysis and psychotherapy in the 13th district of Paris, run at the time by Alain Gibeault; and also at the Bichat Hospital, in a department of gastroenterology where "psychosomatics" had an important place.

The principles that today govern the preliminary interview are, for the most part, those that were adopted in the initial stages of my experience. Some of these principles – such as the renunciation of suggestion – had even been formulated by Freud (1913). It has to be recognised, though, that, remarkably, the way psychoanalysts belonging to one and the same school conduct a preliminary interview can differ significantly. That is why it is important to begin by looking at the theoretical foundations involved.

First, it should be emphasised that the consultation conducted by a psychoanalyst has its own strict specificity; in other words, it is fundamentally different from the psychiatric consultation which takes the medical consultation as its model. That is why, in this psychoanalytic interview, the analyst's personality must, as we know, efface itself as much as possible with a view to preserving the place and role of the analyst as the so-called transference object that the patient, unconsciously, sees in him or her. And even when this model does not fall into place spontaneously and sufficiently, the analyst must respect the necessity of not impeding its development. Let us recall (doctrine and theory require us to do so) that provided that it is rigorously conducted, the purpose of the preliminary interview is to give the patient every chance to react in a ludicrously distorted way, not to the other of reality, but to the object that he/she projects into him or her, a ghost, in fact, an imago. In other words, the interview is "riddled" with the transference. The other in question is part of the question of "thirdness" of which Alain Gibeault speaks. All that is well known, but I will nonetheless give an illustration of it.

A woman patient, aged about 50, evoked in the preliminary interview the severe suffering that had resulted from her relationship of emotional dependence on a woman friend. It was significant that she named this friend by her first name; I will call her Marie. Struck by this detail, I said to her: "You are putting Marie into my arms". This was a "wild" interpretation and, some would say, premature in an interview that revealed both transference and unconscious homosexuality. This introduction swiftly paved the way for what was to be a particularly fruitful analysis. If I am reporting this radical circumstance, it is because, in doing so, and with regard to the position I defend, namely, *a single preliminary interview, and two at the most*, I find I am not in agreement here with Jean-Luc Donnet with whom I had a lengthy discussion on the subject more than ten years ago (Donnet & de M'Uzan, 1998). Sharing the same cultural background as me, Jean-Luc Donnet argued that "the first meeting is not analytic" and advocated – excluding "natural analysands" – the multiplication of preliminary interviews (four, or even six); in this respect, his position was quite close to the Freudian idea of a "preliminary experiment" (Freud, 1913, p. 124).

Clearly, it is a matter of what might be called a strategy of the preliminary interview; an interview, in certain respects, that is comparable to the game of chess, before tactical manoeuvres are involved.

Contrary to my initiative in the case of Marie, the "key" strategic instrument at the analyst's disposal is silence, opening out onto to his or her attribute as a transference object. And I am inclined to think that it is countertransference reactions that impede the implementation of this technical measure.

The technical measure correlative to silence is that of *giving fresh impetus to the associative process* by simply taking up what the patient has said in an interrogative or exclamatory manner, which I combine with the interpretation of a defence, and not of a content, in order to enable the patient to continue speaking. In this way, and while avoiding making an interpretation of content (as I did, nevertheless, in the case of Marie), I reveal a *mode* of functioning of the psychical apparatus, without running the risk of introducing into the psychic space of the patient, and by means of the transference, ideational contents that were not there before and that function like "psychic cysts". Thus we find ourselves responding to requirements of an ethical order. I would add that the analyst's silence plays a part in creating an atmosphere of strangeness, a sign that the problematic of identity has been engaged. Here we are touching on the analyst's power, which is considerable; indeed, it is at the limits of what is acceptable. Not to mention the fact that, from the outset, the role of seduction is posited, and posited seriously, for the technical rigour of which I am speaking exposes the analyst to a very early inscription of the infantile past in the present situation, which cannot escape the notice of the analyst who is aware of the dangers that can easily be imagined. Rather than thinking he or she is sheltered from the risk of seducing the other, would it not be better for the analyst to recognise it, to recognise the weight of the potential desire to do so? Are we not dealing here with a caricature of what occurs in any interpersonal relationship? One may be an analyst, but one is still a human being! Knowing that the technical rigour which I defend, even in the preliminary interview, is liable paradoxically to create an atmosphere of seduction, should make it possible to take responsibility for the fact that we are engaged in a policy of "brinkmanship".

Conducted in keeping with the principles that I have just set out – even if this is not always possible – the preliminary interview acquires the characteristics of a strange and ineffable meeting that is nostalgically inscribed in the patient's memory, and sometimes in the analyst's too. In passing, and parenthetically, we may wonder if the analyst's eventual unconscious complicity does not play a part in bringing about the situation in which certain analyses are completed and yet interminable? However that may be, the meeting between the protagonists ideally takes the form of a *mise en scène* of characters, and not people, as on the stage of a theatre. And when the interview continues to develop in this way, which unfortunately is not always the case, we see what I call a translation of identity asserting itself, whereby the shadow of the imagos covers over that of the real persons. The analyst resists this, more or less unconsciously, because the narcissistic solution found – created by the patient in response to the initial drama – had been effective for a long time. Reactualised in the transference – as we know – this solution is expressed through dramas involving *characters*, but also, and primarily, in *the way in which the psychical apparatus functions*, according to its mechanics, if I may put it like that. That is the essential point, for the *contents* themselves are more or less random and liable to replace each other in the metonymic, and at best symbolic, mode. As a result, the analyst's listening and interventions, which had hitherto been oriented almost naturally towards history, are turned instead towards its motive forces which contributes to aggravating the atmosphere of strangeness I referred to earlier. The analyst's attention, still held by the dramas affecting the analysand, now turns towards his/her problematic of identity. In certain respects, a new path is thus opened up for the analysis of these moments, or of these cases, where what is decisive is the indefinite nature of the frontiers of identity. This situation is infinitely more frequent than one would imagine and calls for a strategic choice whereby the attention focused on the relationship between the sexual and the *vital-identital** (i.e. between the psychosexual and the self-preservative orders) must now be oriented towards the latter, the *vital-identital*. In the very first meeting with the patient, the analyst, ideally, should be able to recognise the state of negotiation between the sexual and the *vital-identital*, for the future of the analysis depends on it.

I have observed the same dramatic evolution of analyses conducted by certain very experienced colleagues on the basis of a diagnosis of obsessional neurosis. One of them was unaware of the order that I call the *vital-identital*, evoked in the last chapter. In this case, the instruments for managing the situation along obsessional lines proved inefficient. The economic dimension began to weigh heavily. As the anal-sadistic regression of the libido was overwhelmed, the situation had evolved and become part of the self-preservative register of identity, namely, the *vital-identital*. Psychosomatically trained analysts are familiar with this evolution.

The analyst, in spite of what one might imagine, by no means always has to deal with morbid entities belonging to the psychosexual order. I have thus noticed a certain development in my views concerning both the analytic treatment itself and its initiation. Briefly, whilst my attention was originally focused on the form taken by the *object-relationship*, I have noticed this relationship shift significantly towards the problematic of identity, towards the recognition not so much of the familiar "no man's land" but of an "every man's land" in which the frontiers of identity of the protagonists dissolve. It will thus not come as a surprise to see me affirming that access to the phenomena of depersonalisation* as well as a capacity for tolerating them are indications of the fundamental psychic disposition required for the psychoanalytic vocation.

Our manner of intervening is not fixed; it evolves in the light of experience. One day, a woman patient arrived dazed and vacillating. She murmured: "I am a hole". There was a time when, hearing these words within a specifically psychosexual register, I would have replied: "I have a hole". On the day in question – quite recently – I replied: "A hole has edges". At the time, analysts were still thinking in terms of the integrative capacities of the preconscious, but new perspectives were opening up.

I thought I would conclude with these lines, feeling that I had now set out the most decisive factors for the analyst when he or she formulates an indication. But that would be to omit matters of routine such as noting the direct questions of the patient in order to possess additional arguments to back up the decision. And so it is by almost giving up this strange identity and slipping in to that of the "doctor", that the analyst, somewhat systematically, asks the patient to tell about a night dream and a memory from early childhood, tokens of his or her capacity for doing analytic work.

Analysis, and of course the preliminary interview, evolve over the course of time, along with the personality of the psychoanalyst, which should come as no surprise. This strange population is not made up of the same sensibilities. Does this play a role in the conduct of the preliminary interview and what follows from it? I cannot help thinking back to the time when, as a young analyst in training, I met the key psychoanalytic figures in France of that era. Among them, I recall Parcheminey, Schlumberger and John Leuba, who had a different relationship to culture. Was it to the point of influencing their technique? I do not know. But I am still perplexed when recalling the memory of a patient, one of Parcheminey's patients, I think, who, at the beginning of his analysis, and out of provocation, would recite during the entire session the stanzas of Horace in Latin. At a certain moment he stopped, and Parcheminey then continued the recitation, also in Latin. It spelt the end of the patient's resistance on that day.

Notes

1 This chapter was first published as a paper in *L'Inquiétude permanente*, pp. 77–82 (de M'Uzan, 2015a).

2 Translator's note: In French *"Qui de moi?"* (lit. "Who of me?"). In less literary terms, "Which part of me?"

Chapter 8

Last words (1981)[1]

On two occasions previously, I have been led to pursue a number of reflections on the theme of death. On the first occasion I dwelt on the fantasy that I called "S.j.e.m." ("*Si j'étais mort*"); on the other, I was essentially concerned with the fate of the libido in the dying person (see de M'Uzan, 1974a, 1976a). I was trying at the time to circumscribe an original psychic activity, in certain respects comparable to the work of mourning, which has considerable importance when one is negotiating the last moments of life.

Today, I want to return to the same theme in order to examine another aspect of it. This work is a result of the analytic interviews that I had with a woman suffering from widespread secondary cancer. I would perhaps not have embarked on it if the patient had not explicitly expressed the wish that something remain of what she had been discovering tragically over a number of weeks, that is, of her need to understand the new states into which she had been plunged. It is clear that her testimony represents the essential part of this work.

***

Mrs D. came to see me at the beginning of November 1977. She told me at the outset that she wanted to have my advice about the possibility of doing a "tranche" of analysis in order to overcome some neurotic symptoms that had been insufficiently resolved during an earlier personal analysis from which she had otherwise derived great benefit. However justified these reasons were, they were only part of what had driven her to seek a consultation; it was not long before she explained to me the other more essential reasons, concerning the evolution of a cancerous illness that had begun more than ten years earlier: she had developed bilateral breast cancer which had required two very mutilating surgical interventions. But in spite of these interventions, the process did not stop; four years before she decided to come to see me, something she had intended to do years before that, disseminated bone metastases had appeared. Their importance was reduced by a combination of radiotherapy and chemotherapy, without, however, eliminating them entirely. The prognosis was thus gloomy. Mrs D. knew this perfectly well, having been informed both of the diagnosis and the metastatic dissemination. Whether the attitude of the oncologist was right or not is certainly debatable; for my part, and in this case particularly, I want to say that telling the truth is the best solution, for it is possible that this "knowledge" mobilised in Mrs D. unsuspected forces that were put in the service of her determination to fight – a tenacious determination attested by the absorbing professional activities that she continued to pursue almost to the end.

In our first interview, and on more than one occasion thereafter, she said to me, as if in passing, that she was sometimes fed up with suffering, that she was so tired that sometimes she was on the point of "giving up". But, she asserted vigorously, her desire to live, and to go on living, was always even stronger. The step she took that day in coming to see me was part of this struggle, a struggle in which, I would add, she had the rare fortune to be helped by the tender, attentive and unfailing presence of her husband.

Having thus put me in the picture, she quickly assured me that she had not come to ask me to help her die. This was true, because she wanted me to help her live as fully and intensely as possible. But her thoughts must have been a bit more ambiguous, since a few days later she acknowledged her fear that I might refuse to enter into the therapeutic relationship that she wished for so keenly. To tell the truth, this fear was not completely unfounded; although I had made a positive decision quickly, I noticed in fact that my listening lacked flexibility, that I was thinking too much. I saw this as the expression of a reticence to take on such an overwhelming problem, as the unacknowledged, if not unconscious, wish to reject the person who had reserved this task for me. In short, it was one of those "countertransference reactions" that I will be discussing in more detail later on.

My attitude, however, did not apparently betray too much of my resistance because Mrs D. did not hesitate to give me more information and to reveal her secret hope. She insisted that she knew that she was very, very ill, invaded by metastases affecting her feet, her spine and the dome of her skull; and she did not know how long she still had to live. She experienced her state as a "chronic and nameless humiliation", and this was what she wanted to repair at the price of a final effort for which she was seeking my assistance. Sensing I would agree, she said to me, rather as one makes a confession, "I am once again involved in a creative process".

The analytic relationship was now underway, but the malignant evolution had unfortunately taken a turn for the worse. New bone metastases soon appeared, then she was in real respiratory distress, indicating that the illness had extended to her lungs; and finally her overall state deteriorated to an alarming extent and her liver was invaded. But, notwithstanding all this suffering, and apart from a short hospitalisation of about three weeks in June 1978, Mrs D. came to her sessions, alone at first, and then accompanied. She came with incredible determination, and continued to do so until three days before her death, at the end of the month of October 1978. It was almost a year since she had come to see me for the first time.

***

Mrs D.'s words, "I am once again involved in a creative process", were reminiscent of a classical function, as it were, of analysis, since anamnesis is not only a matter of recalling one's personal history, but of constructing a new history in which the analyst and the analysand are closely associated. Now Mrs D. did indeed bring me a history in which those famous neurotic residues were rooted and which, for a while, had served her as a screen. This history, moreover, was elaborated easily and quickly in a very condensed form which highlighted the situation of the central character, her mother. She had died during my patient's early childhood and was the object of a variety of feelings that were nonetheless dominated by vigorous hatred. She had "passed on her venom" to her, she said. But this issue had largely been dealt with during her earlier analytic experience, so I shall not dwell on it now, particularly as it was not at all an essential feature of the perspective that was facing me.

During the preliminary interview, Mrs D., let me recall, had stressed the importance that she attached to the fact of feeling involved in a creative process. I was very struck by this. Thereafter, she often referred to the notion of creative activity and to its interference in the work that we were doing. But in this case it was not simply a matter of reconstructing a neurotic history, nor even of a sort of reaction to the fear that she expressed on several occasions of "not being up to it, of lacking resources at the level of fantasy, of feeling she was devoid of imagination and dreams".[2] And I had the intuition that the mention of creativity, which was rather remarkable if one considers what was going on at the vital level, concerned the illness itself, and then the particular psychic activities that would be mobilised in her by her precise knowledge of her state and of its likely fatal outcome.

As I have already said in an earlier paper (de M'Uzan, 1976a), this psychic activity is related to the object relations of the subject who is mortally stricken: a regressive greediness in relationships, a voracious flaming up of desire, a paradoxical expansion of drive activity, etc. But it also affects the ego's relationships with the subject's body, with his/her very being, which for me is not contradictory because I have been led to link the problem in relationships with a wavering of the frontiers between the inside and the outside. "Living, I act and react as a mass; dead I act and react as molecules", Diderot said in a striking turn of phrase, though personally I would hesitate before adopting it wholesale. Being naturally inclined to interest myself in the intermediate regions, in zones of passage, in the area "between dog and wolf", as the French saying goes, I think that between the two states evoked by Diderot, there is room for a transitional space in which the integration of the organism is called into question. But the mechanisms involved in this in-between space do not escape the influence of the psychical apparatus which, on the contrary, spontaneously and without the knowledge of consciousness, tries to give them a direction, to orient them, while at the same time modifying the relations that the subject has both with others and with him- or herself. If this is indeed how things happen, we are justified in speaking of a process by which the last days of any person subjected to the fate of my patient are necessarily determined. More than in everyday life, where it can easily pass unnoticed, it is in the field of the analytic relationship, which very rarely plays a part in such cases, at the heart of the interferences between transference and countertransference, that this process manifests itself most clearly, or even that it is best able to develop itself.

On the subject of the relations between us, I would like to note the extent to which the ambivalence of my patient was expressed abruptly, without nuances, crudely. Hardly had I agreed to follow up on our preliminary interview than the following thought came to her mind: "I hope he doesn't die!" Retrospectively, I realised that this was a profound remark indicating how the morbid phenomena were being cathected. On another day, when, in a peculiar state of euphoria she was inwardly repeating one of my interventions to herself, in order to preserve it, because she thought it was strangely in danger, she suddenly thought about my remark: "He will become shit, like everyone else!" I could cite many remarks of this kind, commonplace remarks, especially as they did not signify an alteration of the confidence that had been placed in me (not to mention the fact that one could easily detect the person at whom the remark was aimed, namely, the mother, whose image reappeared). But the style of this violence was disconcerting, which led me to think that, in the present case, the notion of ambivalence should be reconsidered. I would formulate things as follows: one of the faces of ambivalence is turned towards the past; the other, with which I am chiefly concerned here, is turned towards the future, towards the realisation of a project of which it is one of the instruments. The feelings of love and hate concern a transference object whose identity is always that of an independent subject, recognised as such. On the other hand, alongside what we are familiar with, we can see, at moments and progressively, *affective qualities* partly disappearing in favour of *tendencies* that usually serve them. It is thus no longer a matter of love and hate but of construction and destruction, within a space in which the protagonists are encompassed and swept off their feet to the point that their identity becomes uncertain, and sometimes interchangeable. What is urgent, under these circumstances, is no doubt to thwart the organic fatality but, first and foremost, to ensure the emergence of a new object whose functions are largely unsuspected; an object that participates in this creative activity of which Mrs D. often spoke and which is completely unaware of the particular status of the encompassed objects. Thus, and even when, a moment earlier, the exchange was dominated by the inclination for relationships and the drive expansion that I have described, destroying me or preserving me, entrusting me with a task or annihilating me and annihilating herself along with me became almost equivalent acts. A point was reached when the ordinary register of neurotic exchange was overwhelmed and the state of ambivalence exacerbated, so that the cancer itself then seemed to acquire the status of a protagonist alongside the patient, her body and myself.

One day, when Mrs D. was insidiously multiplying hostile remarks towards me, I said to her quite simply that she was trying to test me. She protested vehemently, saying that for her I was like a "backbone", though her own, she knew, was invaded by metastases! Moreover, she seemed to perceive the deep sense of her words, because she took the initiative of cutting the session short a little ahead of time, "in order to keep you, before you become toxic", she said. A further step was taken when she began to complain more frequently of a feeling of "inner emptiness". This was a long-standing feeling, one, she assured me, that she had always had, a sort of "lack or void that has to be filled". I then felt the need to "give a role" to the cancer and, after an understandable hesitation, I suggested that if this void was not filled by someone, she could fill it herself, and that in her mind her cancer was precisely destined to fill this void. Not without some astonishment on my part, she immediately and vigorously confirmed my intervention, adding that she thought of her cancer as a creation comparable to any other, and even to a pregnancy (she had been pregnant once, but to her dismay had been unable to carry the pregnancy to full term). She remained silent for a moment, as if dreaming, before saying that she had just remembered suddenly that right at the beginning, when her cancer was still developing without her knowing it, she had recalled an infantile fantasy of giving birth via the breast.

A little later on in the analysis, when a sort of rotation of themes had been established, we began again to wonder about the meaning of her cancer, to which I was already ready, personally, to ascribe an identity. It was almost the end of the session. There was a silence. With her dark eyes wide open, my patient stared at me, and time passed. Giving free rein to my thoughts, I thought I could detect in this gaze both the tragic void of a mind that was briefly in a state of arrest and an intense need to absorb me. At the beginning of this same session, and on the subject of one of my interventions, she once again stated: "I must keep that". I now had the feeling that she was taking big swigs of my substance* (see *Psychic aphanasis*) – these were the terms in which I formulated it to myself – while the image of the infant at the breast gazing deeply into its mother's eyes came to my mind. I shall not insist on the countertransferential character of this material, because it is sufficiently clear; but, it is well known, and for my part I have already drawn attention to the fact, that the countertransference is also a tool of understanding, providing an original path of access to what is going on in the patient's mind. Without that, I might have understood Mrs D. less well on the day when, having arrived for her session in spite of everything, she began talking to me in a quietly ironic tone that betrayed intense feelings of superiority. I have experienced a similar situation with a perverse masochist* (see *Masochistic movement*) who, during the interview I was conducting with him, showed himself to be full of pride and defiance (de M'Uzan, 1972).

It is important to understand the significance of this proud and derisive defiance. Could it be the effect of a denial of reality? Not exactly, because reality is recognised and rejected in turns; it is recognised when Mrs D. openly describes what is going to happen to her, and rejected when, making travel plans, she denies the obvious signs of the seriousness of her state. The macabre humour that she readily employs perhaps forms a bridge between these two attitudes. At any rate, this particular form of denial strongly evokes the beginning of a split in the ego. Moreover, I am bound to say that it was not the classical implications of this notion that first held my attention. Indeed, I had the intuition that denial and splitting intervened above all in connection with a major projective process participating in the creative activity dear to my patient.

One day, after I had pointed out the difficulty that Mrs D. had in making links between several memories, and having added that this difficulty no doubt had a role to play in the struggle that she was involved in, she replied that she was very well aware of that. Then, without any transition, she assured me that I could not imagine the ordeal she went through every morning, when she had to "reconstruct herself entirely". She meant this in the strict sense, for she had, in effect, day after day, to put prostheses in the place of her amputated breasts and to put on a wig to hide a total loss of her hair due to chemotherapy. Consequently, it is understandable that she sometimes murmured: "Why continue to struggle when one carries death in oneself?". A spontaneous thought came to my mind: just as one carries a child, which confirmed my impression that a personification of the cancer was taking place. But Mrs D. by no means remained bogged down in what she had just said, it was just a passing moment of depression. She soon rediscovered her energy and returned to her fundamental objective by letting me know that she would have liked me to "descend" into her cancer. This time I did not hesitate any longer and I asked her frankly what the identity of the cancer was, by which I meant, and she understood very well, the identity of this *person*. Somewhat disconcerted, she produced a few associations which, although apparently conventional, nonetheless had the merit of leading her to a name, *Uccelli*, by which she was rather taken aback. The name was completely unknown to her; according to her, the fact that her father was of Italian ancestry had nothing to do with it. "Uccelli", she said, "the name certainly intrigues me, just as your own name intrigues me, yes, indeed!" And while she was about it, she added: "How I would've liked to serve you, for you to be my spokesman, like that I would leave a trace!" To which she added, shortly after, the wish to "fecundate" me in order to survive in me and at the same time to take control of me. Thereafter, the regime of the activities of representation, whose deficiencies she had complained about, began to change: we witnessed a progressive enrichment of the phantasmatic and oneiric functions which developed in parallel in the relational register and in the narcissistic register, the latter of which particularly held her attention. Following my intervention concerning the identity of the cancer, and after this sequence, patient, cancer and analyst became almost interchangeable as images, given that their frontiers were so labile. Over the course of the weeks, these moments of wavering became increasingly frequent, but for my part I saw nothing negative in this. On the contrary, the more we advanced, the more I felt we were dealing with a constructive process oriented towards a precise objective that was matched by a parallel evolution in my countertransference.

To begin with, the countertransference manifestations to which I have referred were, on the whole, quite ordinary. More surprising was the subsequent emergence of unusual images and thoughts, nourished primarily by primary processes and sometimes without any apparent links with the manifest context. I have already given an example above by evoking my patient's gaze. At other moments, it was a matter of vague emotions, verging on moody states. Finally, I had the painful impression that I was missing something, an impression, in fact, that I never completely overcame; it was as if I had come up against an insurmountable material object. In order to illustrate the course of the reflections that I had at the time, which led me to express some rather unclassical ideas on the countertransference, I will now venture to report a brief sequence.

That day a question arose concerning the protocol and rhythm of the sessions. Although our meetings had been taking place regularly for several months, Mrs D. once again raised the issue of this aspect of our work. The organisation of the sessions suited her perfectly; she would have liked to have more, certainly, but it was impossible, etc. She said that in a quiet, measured tone, which suggested to me that there was something behind all this serenity; and once again I had the impression I was missing something. Of course, it is often the analyst's lot to suspect that his or her understanding of the material is insufficient. This time, however, I was persuaded that this was a different experience. I therefore felt the need to dwell on the issue, though without communicating this to my patient. Once again we talked about the theme of the cancer, its evolution and death, all in a tone whose serenity stood in stark contrast to the nature of the subject. And I reflected on this discordance, which seemed to me to be the sign of a sort of shared denial: in short, my patient and I did not want to know anything about what we were talking about.

I immediately associated this theme of denial with that of psychosis; but I then took a step back, telling myself that, in such a context, evoking psychosis in a theoretical mode was nothing more than an attempt to ward off anxiety. While that is true, I then understood that this return of my thoughts about denial and psychosis was hiding another aspect of my countertransference, namely, the need to push away the recent feeling I had been having that I was missing something. Having taken this step, I finally understood that what was missing, was the possibility of assuming full responsibility for a megalomaniac position of omnipotence. It will be said that if analysts get to the point of regretting that they are not mad enough to believe, or not capable of believing, that the full utilisation of primary mechanisms in their therapeutic work can, for example, stop the evolution of the cancer, then that is a peculiar conception of the countertransference! And yet I think that it is almost necessary to reach this degree of madness in order to give every chance to the psychic work that is required by this kind of situation to which my patient had committed all her strength.

This is not the first time that I have expressed ideas of this kind. I have done so in particular in respect of seriously ill psychosomatic patients who taught me how important it is for analysts to be able to tolerate a certain vacillation of the frontiers of their egos in order to be able to receive the deadly contents that their patients are trying to get rid of; and also how important it is for them to be able to accept the strange contact that is established with this type of patient. Whether it is symbolic or concrete, this contact acts as a sort of erotic zone, and the auto-erotic expansion that proceeds from it is a first step towards a new cathexis of the body and its image. It is only then that the image that the subject has of him- or herself, a broken, fragmented and unacceptable image, can be reorganised in favour of another self-image that is still mutilated, to be sure, but better integrated. When, however, as was the case here, a fatal outcome is foreseeable, the problem is quite different from one where it is simply a matter of restoring a self-image that is already repairing itself. The only thing that is common to the two situations is what underpins the analyst's attitude. Finally, I would add that, as in all the cases where the analytic relationship has been properly established, the psychic work that develops in the patient, but also in the analyst, follows a sort of trajectory; that is to say, it goes through several phases and follows a progression which, although it runs parallel to that of the illness involved, is nonetheless distinguishable from it. In the present case, since I was perfectly aware of the situation, I should have detected this trajectory earlier; in fact, I was often caught up in the demands of the moment, and only saw things more clearly as I became aware of the evolution of my countertransference on the one hand, and on noticing the development of my patient's oneiric activities on the other. While she had had very few dreams during the first months, they had now become more and more frequent and concerned the patient's relationship with herself and her own body more than her relationships with her objects. Thus, just before the holidays, she dreamt that she was in pieces and that she was being put together again with earth. But even when the narcissistic organisation seemed to take precedence over the object-directed organisation, the two themes continued to coexist in her, as in every analysand, and they would remain associated until the end. For example, in the previous session, she told me in an ironic tone, as usual, that with all the money that she was giving me she could buy herself clothes to please me (here I am reminded of Janice Norton's patient, whom I have referred to in an earlier paper [see Norton, 1963; cited in de M'Uzan, 1976a; 2013b, p. 37ff.]). She may have said this out of pure bravado, but it was also to do with her determination to live at all costs, a determination that was never really dented, even when she had suicidal thoughts or felt like "giving up". In fact, whenever she thought of putting an end to her life, she mainly wanted to put an end to a humiliating physical condition, and also to underline the bitter struggle that she had to lead to resist the temptation of giving way to passivity.

At the stage of the treatment that I have just been referring to, which revealed some original – I would almost say specific – mental work, I saw two series of themes emerge clearly: on the one hand, seduction, a devouring of the object, and the desire to leave an indelible mark on it; on the other, a denial of reality, an effort of reconstruction and the cancer as creation. But scarcely had I discerned the meaning of this complex organisation than something else seemed to be preparing itself.

During this summer of 1978, it became clear that the point of no return had been reached. The oncologist who was following Mrs D. had apparently even situated it a few months earlier. But, from my own position, the subtle variations of her state, both on the moral as well as the organic level, convinced me that the struggle was continuing in much the same way as at the beginning of our meetings. One could no longer say the same in September; by that point it was obvious that a new phase of the battle had been embarked on. Old themes reappeared, the memory of her mother came back to her, largely free of the ambivalence that had coloured it previously; and this was even true when Mrs D. recalled the pleasure that her mother had taken in trying to have a fusional relationship with her. Spontaneously and calmly, she talked about the connection that she saw between her mother and death, and then the theme of time, which took on increasing importance: "Each minute must be filled", she said to me, adding immediately, "But they are always filled!".

Her levels of fatigue increased, confining her to a state of exhaustion, and she was frightfully short of breath, but in spite of this Mrs D. continued to come. And it was our last meeting. The dry and unremitting cough from which she was suffering so much had diminished somewhat thanks to a drug prescribed by her doctor.

I saw her opposite me, saying, "this time I'm going to die"; she felt like letting herself slip away, but once again she rebelled against this temptation. She remained silent for a moment and then said to me that she was hesitating about whether or not to tell me about a strange phenomenon that she had recently observed. Deciding suddenly that she would, she described it to me in these terms: "You see, it's not me who is ill, it's the other"* (see *Paraphrenic twin*). And she added, with a smile, "No, I'm not schizo, don't think that. It's a matter of something light, barely perceptible, a sensation at my side. How tiresome it is to have something at one's side like that".[3]

***

Defying all reason, the last words of my patient had not prevented me from still hoping for a remission. I did not actually think that it was possible, at such a moment, to conceive so penetratingly and to formulate so concisely what the subject's ultimate relationship with her perishable being can be. In just a few words my patient settled her account with the psychotic dimension of the phenomena she was experiencing, dramatised the other, her other, expelled it and finally got rid of the morbific principle by which she was affected. In a single sentence a considerable amount of psychic work was condensed, and this is what I want to look at now.

Within a global perspective, I will distinguish three essential aspects: a particular vicissitude of the narcissistic libido; the role of projection; and the appearance of the "other", which I shall here call the double. In reality, these three aspects are closely intertwined and form part of an original psychic process, evolving in phases, that is perhaps specific to the final stage of a mortal illness.

I described earlier those aspects of this psychic process that are related to object relations, as they appear in the transference. In this last state they express a deep need to mark the object with an indelible stamp in order to survive in it. This moment constitutes a sort of articulation with the other path taken by the process, namely, the relations of the ego with its own body. Here, too, a series of precise themes can be observed that open out onto the role of denial, which I have already discussed at length in relation to Mrs D.'s attitude and my countertransference movement. But what is the real issue at stake when denial is opposed to the recognition of such a serious organic alteration? However aware or not the subject is of it, any pathological organic malfunction, and no doubt even any somatic activity eluding integrated modes of functioning, is perceived by the psychic apparatus, which then seeks ways to enact them, that is to say to give them meaning in accordance with its synthetic function. But this attempt is far from always successful, particularly in the case of a cancerous dissemination, given the scope and anarchic character of the illness. Faced with the immense narcissistic disappointment that results, denial only offers very provisional recourse, even when it helps preserve a sort of bastion behind which the ego can hide; or even when, being insufficiently active, it associates itself with a search for meaning (cancer "experienced as a creation"). This resides essentially in the particular economic problem raised by an organic malfunction. By approximating hypochondria and organic illness from the point of view of the distribution of the libido, Freud (1914) drew attention to the concentration of libido that occurs in a sick organ. This is an entirely general phenomenon concerning both sick organs and new organs in the form of metastases which are regularly the object of a hypercathexis of narcissistic libido, and even a truly local stasis that naturally goes hand in hand with a substantial modification of the libido invested in the ego. This particular status of the narcissistic libido cannot, it seems, be tolerated for very long and requires a new psychic action to be undertaken, whose primary objective is to evacuate the excessive quantity that is responsible for an unbearable level of "tension". Only projection, which plays a decisive role, is in a position to carry out this task, albeit at the price of a new accentuation of modifications of the ego; for the mechanism is applied at the same time to the patient's own body, a body that may henceforth be considered as split in two because its quasi "twin"* (see *Paraphrenic twin*) half is expelled by the cancer. It is no longer Mrs D. who is ill, it is the other, her double. The feeling of uncanniness that accompanies this projection of the subject's own body belongs, of course, to the sphere of depersonalisation,* but although Mrs D. did indeed feel split in two, it did not reach the point where one could speak of persecution. The double was next to her in the form of a "light" and "barely perceptible" presence that was both unusual and familiar, though without in any way creating anxiety. It was certainly a phenomenon of a hallucinatory character, but Mrs D. did not confer a definite identity on this new being; she did not even seem to know that it was a part of herself. Being external, without playing a persecutory role, sick but alive, the double assumes multiple functions which stem precisely from its paradoxical function. It is what has to die in the place of the patient, and thus what ensures his or her survival; it preserves up to a certain point a sufficient narcissistic cathexis of the subject's being. Contrary to what one might think, it serves to reduce the danger of fragmentation insofar as it is projected as an entity; it may also polarise a new cathexis comparable to an object-cathexis – which would be a "cure", as delusion is in the case of psychosis. But, charged with all the "lethalness", the one that must die is also the one that Mrs D. ought to mourn with the secret hope of achieving, thereby, a final instinctual drive introjection in parallel with that which she carries out in relation to her love-objects, including her transference object.[4]

While the double appears with functions that are relatively easy to imagine, its origin, on the other hand, poses a much more complex problem. And though it stems from a projective mechanism, this particular form of projection can only be understood in relationship with the regression of the ego which is strongly involved here. As for the hallucinatory character of the phenomenon, it indicates the probable level of the regression, for it is comparable to what happens when the human infant (Tausk, after Freud, showed this clearly) does not yet have the possibility of forming a conception of memories as such, but discovers them in the outside world in the form of things seen, existing in reality. In this sense, it can be argued that independently of its level, the idea of the spread of secondary cancers participates directly in the appearance of the double by "opening up" the path for projection. It is as though it followed a schema of splitting that had existed almost forever in the image that the patient had of herself.

By expelling her double* (see *Paraphrenic twin*) into a space separate from her own, Mrs D. was ensuring that a part of herself had a status of extraterritoriality comparable to that which exists in the first stages of life, when the body, which is strictly speaking not inhabited, is still largely an object to be discovered and cathected. The double of the end may be said to proceed, therefore, from that of the very first beginnings, whose fate is to plunge into the shadows and to lead a secret existence there that only certain events are capable of revealing. However, this retrograde movement operates less as a defensive mechanism in the common sense of the term than as what, at a given moment, enables the individual to discover him- or herself as in the most archaic times of being ("*s'anté-découvrir*"). The conjunction of projection and regression leads the dying person to lose the habit of recognising the alter ego that he or she has constituted as being part of him- or herself. At the end of life an individual is sent back to what I shall call the *zone of individuation* beyond which a truly integrated existence begins, and prior to which the fragmented body does not belong to the child any more than the child's first thoughts do.

It was by linking the expulsion of the double to a projection of the body itself that I was struck by the analogy between the process that I have described and that presented by Victor Tausk (1919) in his study "On the Origin of the 'Influencing Machine' in Schizophrenia". The thesis is well known: the machine, forged by delusion, is mysteriously linked to the schizophrenic whom it persecutes in every way possible. As a late manifestation of a process that goes through several stages (sense of alteration, then alienation and finally persecution), the apparatus manipulated by enemies is the result of a projection of the patient's own body. For Tausk, the phenomenon results from a regression towards a very archaic stage "when the whole body is a genital organ", or towards that moment when the projection of the subject's own body is a defence against a position of the libido corresponding to the end of foetal development and the beginning of extra-uterine life.

The double of my patient and the "influencing machine" surely have something in common, since in both cases the regression goes back to the sphere of development where "the infant discovers that his own body is fragmented and part of the outer world". Resulting in both cases from a regression and a projection, the apparatus and the double have a very similar economic function; and they also have in common an evolution through phases and a fundamentally narcissistic objective. But the analogy stops there: with Mrs D. the process does not go beyond a sense of alteration, and then of transformation with hallucinatory projection. You will recall that she was not disturbed by her double, and in no way persecuted as the psychotic can be.[5] Her *alter ego* was not an inanimate thing manipulated from the outside, but a ghost which, if it did not have life, at least had the appearance of it. As for localising the period to which the phenomena that I observed related, I would hesitate to do so as precisely as Tausk. Unless he was thinking of a more extended period, to which I would readily subscribe, just as I agree with his idea that inner and outer events never cease to occur, compelling people to constantly rediscover their beginnings. There is one point that remains to be examined, in the nature of a conjecture: could the double, just like the influencing machine, represent the sexual apparatus extended to the whole body? This cannot be excluded, owing to the role attributed to the phallic image in a devastated narcissistic economy, but I find it difficult to say any more about that.

***

Having reached the end of these considerations, and also because nothing ever seems guaranteed, we may ask ourselves once again if the analytic relationship substantially helped my patient fulfil her wish to live fully until the end, if it was really what contributed to the "creative process" on which she hoped she had embarked by the end of our first interview. Mrs D. was convinced this was so, and so was I, especially if I think back to the sequence of the different phases of the treatment right up until the last words that inspired me to write this paper.

But what strikes me now is that, on the point of concluding, I see new hypotheses presenting themselves to me, which, one day perhaps, I will have to put to the test. Consider, for instance, the idea of traversing, *against the flow of time*, this phase in which the human being is born a second time while unifying him- or herself; and that of the discovery of psychic activity which, taking up an existence that is practically void of personal experiences, is concerned with this other moment when all personal experiences are in the process of becoming meaningless: both ideas raises the question of the origin of the mental functions involved or of the psychical apparatus that is at work in this situation. Does the retrograde movement impose a deconstruction of certain functions in the hope of rediscovering an archaic psychical apparatus? Or is it conceivable that as death approaches this archaic apparatus becomes active again under the pressure of a fantasy that has been present since the very first phases of life, namely, the fantasy of the double* (see *Paraphrenic twin*)? But should this fantasy itself not be linked to something that precedes it, to a sort of "hollow representation" destined to be filled by the demands of evolution more than under the pressure of an event?[6] If that were the case, the fantasy of the double would be comparable to the primal fantasies, and the dying person, having expelled the double, would concern him- or herself with origins in order to organise the last hours of life.

Notes

1 This chapter was first published in 1981 as a paper in the *Nouvelle Revue de psychanalyse*, 23, pp. 117–130. It was reproduced in *La Bouche de l'inconscient*, Paris, Gallimard, 1994.

2 These traits form part of a form of mental functioning characterising the psychosomatic structure. Usually, they are associated with a mental activity called "operational thinking" (*pensée opératoire*).* This activity, which was very poorly represented in the case of my patient, is related to conscious processes; it refers essentially to the present which it reduplicates and describes without really signifying the action in process. On this subject, see Marty and de M'Uzan (1963).

3 Having become acquainted with this paper, my colleague Dr Émile Pernin told me what he had observed during his last visit to a patient suffering from lung cancer. The episode occurred less than twenty-four hours before the patient's death. Dr Pernin found his patient lying on his bed and suffering from extreme respiratory distress. It was summer time, and Dr Pernin was standing a few steps away from him near to a large open window. In a voice that was apparently intact, and as if feeling sorry for someone, the patient said to him: "You have seen how this man is suffering and has difficulty . . .". Dr Pernin had the impression that his patient was suddenly very close to him, and he heard him add, "even though we are so very close to the window".

4 For me, the Ego is not only built on the basis of its identifications, but also thanks to their liquidation which occurs through a series of experiences of real or symbolic mourning. While these experiences of mourning lead to the classical incorporation of the lost-object, this only constitutes a preparatory stage for an attempt to introject the instinctual drives invested in the said object.

5 I should add, however, that in a similar case, delusional persecutory themes developed right at the end.

6 Laplanche and Pontalis seem to follow a similar direction of thought in their 1964 article "Fantasme originaire, fantasme des origines, origine du fantasme".

Chapter 9

The mouth of the unconscious (1978a)[1]

I would like to make one remark to begin with: nowadays, anyone who ventures to speak about therapeutic implications in psychoanalysis is liable to be mocked; it is no longer fashionable. As for the term "cure", only a candid mind can allow itself to utter it. In spite of that, the excluded term often returns, and analysts are then quick to sneer, adding an adjective to it that modifies its meaning. Thus connoted, the notion of cure may have been considered as the stigma of some horrible destiny: the outcome of a process of subjection. And yet these therapeutic implications form part of the very definition of psychoanalysis. So what is the origin of this evolution? Was it foreseeable from the beginning? Undoubtedly, at least up to a certain point, because Freud never failed to draw attention to the ambiguities of the notion of cure, as well as to the uncertainties of the process that was supposed to lead to it. Thus, in "Analysis Terminable and Interminable" (Freud, 1937), he points out, on the subject of our "therapeutic efforts", that the patient's ego may experience recovery as a new peril and therefore bring into play a resistance against the uncovering of resistances. Further on, in the same text, Freud links the "force that is absolutely resolved to hold on to illness and suffering" (p. 242) first to the sense of guilt and to the need for punishment, that is, to the ego's relation to the superego, and then to an immanent masochism functioning "beyond the pleasure principle" that can be traced back to the "original death instinct of living matter" (p. 243). Admittedly, this was in 1937, but it is important to note that Freud's scepticism, or even pessimism, had been expressed well before this. In his paper "Lines of Advance in Psycho-Analytic Therapy" (1919a [1918]), he denounced the negative implications of the patient's progress, affirming that every improvement in his condition "reduces the rate at which he recovers and diminishes the instinctual force impelling him towards recovery" (p. 163). For Freud, the improvement obtained by virtue of the mobility of the libido encourages the patient to create new substitutive satisfactions in the place of symptoms which are devoid of the feature of suffering, and which lead to a loss of time, acting out or even organic illnesses. Ultimately, the patient may even look for substitutive satisfactions in the treatment itself, which would justify increasing the atmosphere of frustration, perhaps the introduction of active techniques, and would encourage the analyst, in any case, to give up therapeutic ambition (1912, p. 119). In fact, Freud's cautious reservations concerning the strict success of analytic treatments, and thus the possibilities of curing patients, had been expressed much earlier. Traces of this can be found in a letter to Wilhelm Fliess dated 16 April 1900 (see Masson, 1985, pp. 408–409). In connection with an analysis that he had just finished, and in spite of the persistence of a number of residual symptoms, Freud wrote: "the apparent endlessness of the treatment is something that occurs regularly and is connected with the transference" and that the "asymptotic" conclusion of the treatment "makes no difference to me". But it would be a crude falsification of Freud's thought to assert, as is often done, that it is possible, or even desirable, to remain insensitive to the onslaught of suffering that one sometimes witnesses without being concerned in any way by the most serious eventualities. No, I am even inclined to believe that the most ferocious adherents of a sort of purism according to which all that counts is an ultimate encounter with desire, whatever the consequences, experience something quite different "in practice". Their language is above all the expression of a megalomaniac reaction to the narcissistic wounds inflicted so often on the analyst by the exercise of his or her art.

I think, therefore, that for Freud, as for the majority of analysts, therapeutic concern and scepticism are inseparable. These two extreme positions must be combined, in keeping with the requirements of our practice. It is only by recognising the indissoluble character of this combination that we are justified in pursuing our inquiries into the question of cure or recovery.

***

The best model for cure can be found in the domain of internal pathology. An example is acute lobar pneumonia, as it is called. It generally follows a progression towards a complete recovery, a restitution *ad integrum*. Without this reparation, this healing that leaves no traces or consequences and involves, for the whole organism, a return to the earlier state, one could not speak of cure. Cure does exist then, but we must not forget that even in internal medicine it is never more than the result of an ideal evolution, in short, something that is quite rare. Indeed, if we study conditions that are more or less chronic, we observe facts that are not dissimilar to those we come across in our analyses. The disappearance of symptoms is sometimes achieved without too much difficulty, but in spite of that there is no reason to feel reassured because it is by no means exceptional, far from it, to see harmful consequences of this "cure" appear before too long. For example, new disturbances that develop subsequently; in general, they are more serious than the first and are not unconnected with the effects of a regression. Consequently, somatic symptoms can no longer be considered simply as something bad that needs to be eliminated, or even as the expression of some sort of aggression or other disturbance that needs to be identified. It is important not to overlook the eventual adaptive value of these symptoms, in other words, their economic function. Furthermore, the experienced therapist always wonders about the economic consequences of the lifting of symptoms and about the possibilities of new organisations that may become available to the organism. The therapist also knows that the disorders affecting this or that system sometimes stem directly from a reparation process that could be impeded by untimely interventions.

There exists, then, a certain parallelism between the analyst's ways of understanding symptoms and the doctor's, provided the latter accepts that it is necessary to make a close critical examination of his or her practice and ways of thinking. To be honest, some doctors have taken this sort of examination so far – too far perhaps – that, like analysts, they sometimes begin to call into question the legitimacy – and ultimately the moral legitimacy – of their therapeutic efforts.

Alongside these similarities, there is nonetheless a fundamental difference, which has decisive consequences, concerning the problem of cure. In medical pathology, the aim, whatever one says, is always to *restore an earlier state* that is better and akin to a state of non-illness that is supposed to have existed. Even if it has been "secreted" by the subject him- or herself, illness occurs at a given moment, altering a situation that one would like to be able to restore. Thus, even when one is looking forwards towards a fortunate outcome, that is towards the future, one is necessarily looking backwards: reflection is "retrograde". In analysis, things present themselves quite differently. The point of view, so to speak, is forward-looking, since the objective implicitly proposed is that what was only potential should become actual, that a freedom that was only virtual should assert itself, in short, that *what has never existed should establish itself*. Admittedly, the analyst may be led to scale down the extent of theoretical expectations; in such cases, what he or she is doing is not so much an analysis, in the strict sense, as *analytic work*, which, moreover, is often fruitful. It is no longer possible to speak of cure, even though it is here, precisely, that the therapeutic implications are often the most compelling. Otherwise the term must be placed between inverted commas; ironically, it is all the more acceptable in that at the outset therapeutic concerns were the least compelling factor! But it is necessary to possess a notion and a term, however insufficient they may be, in order to designate an objective, which, for its part is precise: the culmination of an evolution, the outcome of a process that ends with the concretisation of potentialities that the neurotic organisation, notwithstanding its value, would have suffocated.

Before continuing, and in order to clarify my thinking on this topic, I want to recall briefly the ideas I set out in "Transferts et névrose de transfert" (de M'Uzan, 1966). In this paper I cited a text in which Ferenczi asserted that analysis was not an endless process and that it could be conducted until it reached a natural end. I added that every analyst had had the experience on more than one occasion of terminating an analysis with the feeling that this end was logical and, what's more, definitive. In these cases, the entire process, that is to say, the transference neurosis, describes a sort of trajectory whose path is not unrelated to the model that I defined earlier, leading towards a term that was perhaps foreseeable at the beginning of the analysis. "Cure", in the sense I mean it, is identified with the resolution of the transference neurosis, which tends, so to speak, spontaneously towards its extinction by completing "the imperfect denouement of the infantile period". But it is well known that things do not always unfold like this. Sometimes, in fact, the transference neurosis *does not establish itself*. In its place, we see the development of unorganised transferences of affects and emotional stirrings in which we can never identify the role of a third party and which are dominated by covetousness* (see *Egg-laying, covetousness, domination*) demands and need. In this case, the analytic work is just as likely to become interminable as it is to be broken off at any moment.

Insofar as it sets in at a certain moment and then deploys itself until it is finally resolved, the transference neurosis strongly evokes a comparison with a tale whose conclusion also opens out on to a future in which, in principle, everything that destiny had hitherto put on standby is concretised. I would also add that the comparison is all the more legitimate in that the internal structures of the transference neurosis and of the tale are very similar. In both cases, the exchanges between the two protagonists never take place directly, but always with reference to at least one third term. Mediation is thus the rule, while the events are regularly interpreted and falsified. In the transference neurosis, the lived and related history has taken the place of history itself; that is to say, what is said is never an account of a succession of recorded facts as such. Past reality is certainly not wiped out, but rather reorganised and transformed into a "written" past,* oriented by castration and deposited in what I shall call a *meta-memory* from where, potentially, it can be recovered. Marked by fruitful moments, this process has probably never ceased to pursue its course since the distant times of childhood. The elaboration of this past is indispensable in order to constitute a truly repressed dimension that confers on the events, or on the related groups of events, the capacity to be both past and present, that is to say still alive. Elsewhere the ideational material, fixed by a sort of primordial anti-cathexis without a future, remain encapsulated, isolated, incapable of entering into a network of associations.

It could be said that I have simply contrasted two psychic organisations in order to assign them quite different prognoses. That is true, at least in part, for we must not underestimate the specific capacities of certain structures to evolve where a priori one would not have expected it. But I have something else in mind. In the analytic situation, the analysand and the analyst are not simply two characters involved in sometimes difficult relations with each other – relations impregnated by violent affects whose uncertainties often leave their mark on analyses for a long time, and whose resolution is supposed to coincide with the end of the treatment. The analysand and the analyst thus form a sort of new organism, a monster as it were, a *psychological chimera*,* which has its own modes of functioning. Owing to the very nature of the conditions of their encounter, the analysand and the analyst have unwittingly given birth to a fabulous child, a powerful being that operates in the shadows, but whose growth can be more or less affected by all the influences coming from its creators. Among them I have already mentioned those that are related to the analysand's structure. But we must also take into account those that depend on the analyst. I am, of course, not referring to the analyst's knowledge or even know-how, but to something that has to do with his or her mental functioning. The analyst's activity develops at several levels and in different modes. Among them, there is one that differs entirely from the others. Almost at complete variance with the regime that governs waking life, it resembles, without being identical to it, the dream, from which it borrows its principal mechanisms. Analysts, however, can only gain access to this mode of functioning when they are able to tolerate a certain vacillation of their identity, when they can stay in the zone where the frontiers between the ego and not-ego are more than uncertain, when they have preserved a special disposition for primary identification and can tolerate experiences of depersonalisation.* This particular "availability" of the analyst permits the analysand, by means of his or her ideational activity, to invade the analyst's psychic space and to trigger in it the original mental processes that I have previously called paradoxical thoughts* (see *Paradoxical system*) (de M'Uzan, 1977, p. 164). These thoughts, which belong to the analysand, or rather are a potential in him or her, are nonetheless forged in the analyst. More precisely, they depend on the activity of a real system, that which is specific to the *chimera* and which can be placed on the frontiers of the unconscious and the preconscious. The activity of the system manifests itself initially in the form of a procession of ordinary or strange images which occupy entirely, and for a limited period of time, the analyst's mental space. These images – unknown or monstrous faces, distorted landscapes, abstract forms, etc. – merge with each other or are transformed at a regular rhythm, as if in slow motion, through the displacement of their lines and the alteration of their contours, while verbal thoughts, equally unusual, intertwine with these moving forms. Images and enigmatic propositions finally fade into a sort of "cross-fading" when the prevalence of the order of consciousness and external perceptions asserts itself again. All these bizarre forms, at once dense and blurred, circulate constantly and their force can be sensed intuitively. Proceeding from each other and merging with each other, I see them constituting a sort of *fertile magma, a psychological soup* comparable to a fermentable humus, the basis of all genesis the ultimate state of which may be a work of art. If the energy of the paradoxical system comes from the analyst, its matter, in any case, belongs to the *chimera*. The analyst is not powerless with regard to the development of the phenomenon; in particular, he or she can interrupt it. But, as a whole, the analyst lets things follow their course unless too much anxiety arises, which can happen because, in such moments, the analyst finds he or she is "outside" him- or herself.[2]

With the notions of magma, chimera and paradoxical thoughts subject to all the influences stemming from the unconscious and preconscious of the analyst and analysand, we are a long way from the structured narrative, ordered like a tale by castration, which, in my view, characterises the transference neurosis. True enough, the transference neurosis takes up once again, in order to repeat it, the mutation that once took place when the infantile neurosis was establishing itself. But, at the same time, and underneath the manifest symptoms of the transference neurosis, the repressed ideational material that feeds it have maintained special links with other more elementary images that are less organised in relation to each other, "deeper", and more identifiable in part, at least, with primordially repressed material. The paradoxical system opens out onto this region of the unconscious, and it is there that the information that flows in from all sides is initially processed. Furthermore, the *paradoxical system*,* a transitional area, gives original access, from below, to the repressed itself which is thus linked up with the most archaic elements of the unconscious.

I am thus inclined now to consider the transference neurosis from another angle. I no longer see it simply as an ordered reprise of infantile conflicts and as a substitute for the clinical neurosis, but as a construction built, in part, on, and out of, the *chimera** (see *Psychological chimera*), where the unconscious minds of the analysand and the analyst interpenetrate and mingle. The analyst, therefore, is not solely the dedicatee and the agent provocateur of the transference neurosis, but an organic element of its elaboration, for it is in him or her, as if he or she were the analysand him- or herself, that a significant part of the work takes place.

It would be fitting to make a more thorough study of the specific activities that develop on the frontiers of the unconscious and of the preconscious, in that area where the chimera is born. For the time being, I shall simply point out that it is there that a first confrontation occurs between what is most individual in each one of us, instinctual drive presentations, and the external world represented by words. It is in this area that the analyst's unconscious is most fully engaged; a whole chunk of therapeutic activity is decided there.

Our interpretations undoubtedly form an essential part of our task. But as they consist, by definition, of verbal material linked to consciousness, their enunciation takes a certain amount of time, which places them inevitably within a temporal framework, even if, in making them, we have drawn on primary mechanisms, such as condensation* (see *Interpretation*). But alongside interpretations, attention has often been drawn to the role of nonverbal factors in the therapeutic process. Emphasis has been placed on the importance of the tone of voice in which the analyst intervenes, voice inflections, and silence which certainly plays an equally important role. But what I have in mind here is not the absence of speech, the silence of waiting, or the silence that is provoked by anxiety, perplexity or even boredom, whose relations with time are closely interwoven, namely, an unending silence. The silence I am referring to does not have the same relationship with time; I would even say that it is atemporal. It is experienced more as a state concerning which I would readily use spatial references, as if it involved an expanse: an immense silence. In this *fundamental silence** (see *Silence of the psychoanalyst* in the glossary), consciousness does not tense up, it becomes clouded; the usual reference points become blurred and the ego loses itself because it is overwhelmed by the world of images I was referring to earlier, access to which is normally only gained through dreams. It is these characteristics that lead me to say that the analyst's *fundamental silence* has more to do with the principles that govern the unconscious than with those that govern the other psychic systems. *The analyst's silence is the mouth of his or her Unconscious*. It is an opening that gives access to the Unconscious. It is in this silence that the paradoxical system* develops and where the chimera is formed that serves as a starting point for the transference neurosis. In the fundamental silence, excitation tends to follow a *reverse or backward path*, which is expressed by the hallucinatory aspect of the figures that appear in gusts, as it were, when paradoxical functioning is operative.

In order to clarify my thinking, I have already had recourse on one occasion to a biological model (de M'Uzan, 1977). In the same spirit, I shall venture here a reference to physics.

Since, in the unconscious, processes are "timeless", "are not ordered temporally . . . have no reference to time at all" (Freud, 1915, p. 187), we are entitled to say that they occur according to a *negative entropy*, a negentropy, the physical expression of which we are familiar with. Are they not similar to the famous "black holes", whose existence was affirmed because it was necessary theoretically, and one of which at least was identified in the constellation of Cygnus?[3] Whilst, according to the law of increasing entropy that governs our common physical universe, the quantity of information decreases, energy degrades and disorder sets in, according to the law of decreasing entropy, which may be considered as the law of the *conservative* Unconscious, information is constantly accumulating in the silence of the analyst, where it acquires the status of unconscious memories ready to be organised for use in new constructions. And this fundamental silence in which the analyst gathers and retains all the messages coming from the Unconscious, and especially from the patient's, is, in my view, the active agent in the process of cure or recovery.

It is said that recovery involves remembering. Undoubtedly, but on the condition that all the messages, all the events, have been deposited in an *integral memory*, as conceived by information theory. Now is it not a common experience for the analyst to see an earlier thought or something the analysand had said many years before come again to mind? When this happens a work of association begins automatically, as if outside the analyst's mind, but which culminates in a construction that can be formulated in secondarised language. Sparing memories the wear and tear of time, the analyst's silence is thus deeply linked both to the Unconscious and to memory, both of which are governed by negative entropy. Recovery involves remembering, retrieving, but also ordering what had been experienced and forgotten, even if not excluded, so that an evolution interrupted by destiny or neurosis can continue its course. But as soon as this construction is on the point of being completed, entropy is fully empowered again and dispersion begins. Can "cure", however perfect it is, ever be anything other than ephemeral, the expression of a fleeting state? Probably, but it would nonetheless be a triumph of Eros, if it is true that the aim of Eros is indeed to "establish ever greater unities and to preserve them" (Freud, 1940, p. 148), which would not be possible, precisely, without the accumulation of information within a system that is *not subject* to entropy. Contrary to what Freud said, the "fable imagined by certain poets" that living substance was once a unity which had later been torn apart and was now striving again towards reunion, may still have several lessons to teach us.

Notes

1 This chapter was first published in 1978 as a paper in the *Nouvelle Revue de Psychanalyse*, 17, 89–98. It was republished in de M'Uzan, 1994b, pp. 33–44.
2 Translator's note: In French *en deçà ou à côté de lui-même*, lit. short of or at the side of himself.
3 See Charon (1977). When a star has burnt up its combustible matter and is ready to "die", it curls up into itself at the same time as its density increases considerably. From being a "white dwarf" it becomes a "pulsar" whose density

is enormous. The gravitational collapse on its surface conditions a progressive curvature of space which can close in on itself. This is how "black holes" are formed out of which another universe emerges in which the spatio-temporal data are inverted, that is to say, physical phenomena "go back in time": they unfold according to a law of *decreasing entropy*. See also the behaviour of "Maxwell demons" discussed by Jacques Monod (1970) in his book *Le hasard et la nécessité*.

Chapter 10

Interpretation and memory (1993)[1]

Ever since the initial sense of disillusionment due to therapeutic failures, especially at the beginning of the 1920s – failures that were in part at the origin of various doctrinal reorientations, or even acts of dissidence – questions bearing on the deep motive forces of interpretation, and on the mechanisms at work in it, have greatly occupied analysts' minds. They are far from having been resolved, if indeed they ever will be, with regard to the "total psychic activity" of interpretation.* There is every reason, therefore, for continuing to explore the subject. In doing so we find we are constantly faced with ideas, hypotheses and constructions that force themselves upon us, attract us, make us dream, or, conversely, and almost simultaneously, trigger a need to exclude them in the name of this or that rational requirement. At any rate, these ideas soon present themselves to our minds and a remarkable situation then occurs. We notice that the most theoretical reflections, the most abstract thoughts, seem, at some point in their development, to behave like strange interpretations that have emerged from goodness knows where and escape from the analyst's mind, out of defiance perhaps. In this case, interpreting or speaking of interpretation, boils down almost to the same thing. We must therefore preserve both these ways of working when their respective contributions are of value. I would even add that possibilities for theoretical reflection are greatly enhanced when we can apply to them what, in the clinical domain, I call the rule of "as if/like that"* ("*comme si, comme ça*"). When analysts interpret what their patients say, whether it is a matter of dreams, memories, slips of the tongue, etc., they are readily affirmative and say: "Things happened *like that*". It may seem surprising to subject theoretical reflection to this way of thinking; however, I not only consider that it is legitimate to do so, but also, in certain respects, rational. There is a famous saying to the effect that we are entitled to dream provided that we take our dreams seriously.

These remarks directly concern the situation in which I find myself as I return to the question of interpretation. Naturally, I shall follow up the reflections that I have already developed on the subject. The points that held my attention previously were: the economy of interpretation, the sequence of the phenomena that unfold in analysts' minds during the sessions, the mental "risk" that analysts take when an alteration of their sense of identity occurs and finally the nature of the therapeutic action (see de M'Uzan, 1983a, 1983b, 1988, 1991). I want now to take up the question from a different angle.

Analysts know from experience that as their practice becomes more extensive and their reflection deepens, they notice that they are inclined to take greater account of the fact that this or that interpretation was given without having been "thought through" beforehand, and independently of any truly purposeful decision. Shortly after, somewhat dubitative, they say to themselves: "But have I not already formulated this interpretation? In any case, at some point I must have said something similar". The interpretation, then, had already existed before, perhaps in a different form, and it had evolved. Could it have been snatched up and dragged under, as it were, before leading an underground existence that only manifests itself in momentary and unexpected troubling questions? One would like to think that the interpretation, protected by repression and sheltered from the analysts' judgement, had continued to evolve. Under these conditions, the analysts; participation in the phenomenon is neither direct nor deliberate; nor are they the exclusive agent of it. In one sense, one could compare what is happening with the formation and development of the transference neurosis conceived, in part, as the child of that strange being, the "*chimera*",* forged by the merged unconscious minds of the analyst and the analysand (see Chapter 9, "The Mouth of the Unconscious").

Analysts' knowledge and experience, their aptitude for making use of their own emotional reactions to the transference, their capacity to regress while retaining sufficient access to non-symbolic language, certainly enable them to get in touch with their patient's unconscious wishes, to recognise the interference of the past in the present, to detect the presence of desire in defence and guilt, and to identify castration anxiety in transference love, and so on. But it should be acknowledged that these characteristics of a flexible and efficient technique, these agents of a "moved" understanding of unconscious psychic processes, these factors in the discovery of meaning in non-meaning, only reveal a part, albeit an essential part, of the underground evolution of interpretation. Such a movement is sometimes initiated in the first session, or even in the preliminary interview, and gives the impression that one has arrived at a perfect understanding of the situation. And then, whether real or dreamed, the first idea that derives from this understanding is, as it were, dissolved before appearing again later, in a slightly different form, awakening the effect of something "already said" to which I was referring earlier.

Another perplexing factor is the disparity between interpretations of the same material that occurs so often during our discussions. The diversity of the theoretical or doctrinal options is often given as an explanation for this; consider how two interpretations may differ depending on whether priority has been given to a tactical or strategic approach to the text. Mention is also made of the role played by the analyst's personality, by his or her countertransference position when speaking, as well as by the level of listening. It is alleged that the factors involved in understanding are very varied, ranging from those that are the most rational to those that pertain to intuition. These explanations are undoubtedly justified, but they seem insufficient to me because they only apply to one level of mental activity. In my view, another essentially different factor is operative, further "upstream" in relation to the psychic processes described, in determining choices and resolving alternatives.

In order to guarantee, as far as possible, the chances of this hypothesis, it seems to me that it is necessary, in the first instance, to re-examine interpretation as it appears in our practice.

There will be no difficulty in recognising that interpretation cannot be considered in isolation and that it is always the outcome of a specific activity that extends over a long period. Each interpretation proceeds, in fact, from those that have been given before, sometimes in a very different context, but whose cathexis has been maintained. This is how a sort of network is formed in which each interpretation aims to have more than one precise effect. In other words, when analysts intervene, they do more than translate into another language what their patients have just expressed: without doing so deliberately, they exploit the past and forge the future, since each interpretation acquires in turn a preparative function.

In certain respects, an interpretation of the patient's present statements (which is necessarily conservative because it bears the marks of its past), even if it avoids being tyrannical, does actually exclude other interpretations that may be pertinent but which do not impose themselves with sufficient force at that moment. In this way, the current analytic construction is organised at the price of eliminating everything which, albeit conceivable in a different context, is in this instance merely waste material. The interpretation is the "daughter", so to speak, of those that permitted its emergence, but proves to be intolerant of its potential "sisters". In other words, it affirms its will to be the *only one* amongst several others. It is worth noting in passing that certain situations said to be "chaotic" might depend on the loss of this quality.

An interpretation evolves in different but homogenous forms, while gaining a higher degree of specification at each stage. This process, however, is not regular. The analyst often notices that analytic treatment presents alternations, which are difficult to foresee, between periods when interpretive activity accelerates and becomes denser, and periods when it seems to enter a sleeping mode. During this period of stagnation, the effects of an interpretation tend to be scattered because nothing is able to support what is essential or renounce what is of secondary importance. Sometimes, on the contrary, certain "strong" interpretations, expressed in a form that is economically adapted to the situation of the moment, suddenly emerge without apparently owing anything to the process of working-through. Such interpretations create a situation of danger, yet at the same time help the patient to overcome it. But it is rare, though not exceptional, for a psychic "mutation" to occur in such cases. If it happened, it would not only be due to a gain in insight resulting from the combined powers of a change in the psychic economy and a displacement of the ego's frontiers, but also a product of the fact that everything that had been acquired with difficulty had been preserved and even consolidated. But there is something paradoxical here because interpretation, which guarantees something "new" that is favourable and dynamic, must maintain its selective function. To this end, several tactical choices are available to the analyst. One, a very political choice, is for the analyst to content him- or herself with suggesting a meaning on the condition of strongly rejecting this or that other interpretation whose place is indirectly kept in reserve. This generally happens in the analyst's mind, saying to the self before intervening: "I am thinking of this and, above all, not of that". Following another, more brutal, choice, the analyst's interpretation does not result from a debate, but functions selectively, without nuances, eliminating, perhaps wrongly, any version that does not seem to be able to offer sufficient benefit. It could then be said that interpretation *kills* interpretation. Evidence of this is at hand when (and this is far from being a rare situation) an earlier interpretation subsequently comes back to the analyst's mind. The analyst then says to him- or herself: "It would've been better to say nothing; by intervening, I rejected unwittingly what I might have said, the relevance of which is clear to me now. Chance – is it really a matter of chance? – will one day remind me of the eliminated idea, but it may be too late because something essential will have been destroyed. Unless, that is, endowed with a new identity and assuming another role, I can dream the unsaid . . . and, why not, the 'too much said', thereby giving life back again to a shadow that has disappeared and whose fate escapes me".

These remarks lead me to mention a remarkable episode, such as may be encountered from time to time. This episode occurred during an analysis that had been going on for quite a long time and that provided food for thought in more than one respect.

The patient, a teacher and high-level researcher, had been suffering almost as long as she could remember from a symptom that was spoiling her existence: giving her weekly course, something she had been doing year after year, was a source of nagging anxiety. Two days before, she would start accumulating a huge amount of material, fearing that when the time came she would have nothing to say. We are familiar with such neurotic situations but, in this case, and even for an informed observer, the matter was rather surprising, given the experience, knowledge and culture of my patient. Her description of what happened during these moments of suffering was striking. It was difficult not to pay particular attention to this, even when the other things that she said were worthy of interest in more than one respect. The symptom, which the patient often took as the starting point for the things she said in the session, had been analysed and reanalysed in all its accessible forms in the different contexts of the present and the past, as well as in connection with the transference and with a dream. The roles of masochism, repressed exhibitionism, the support of resistance, etc., had been demonstrated in a lively and convincing way, both for the patient and for me. At the same time, I often noted that, within one and the same session, she showed increasing interest in the work she was doing. And yet all this was in vain; the symptom persisted just as before. Coloured by a certain pessimism, as one may well imagine, the patient's fidelity in no way diminished. Equally, my listening was not affected by the slightest lassitude. But I was sometimes astonished nonetheless to see that, in spite of the failure I was experiencing, I still had a lively interest in the story that was unfolding before my eyes. And things continued in this way from week to week and over a period of several months until, one day, somewhat to my surprise, I heard myself express out loud a very personal reflection concerning the work that had been done without any result; indeed, the whole network of interpretations, which were no doubt pertinent, had been put together for nothing. In a half-dreamy, half-meditative tone, I blurted out these words: "And yet it should have worked!" The singularity – it is the least that can be said – of this initiative seemed initially only to arouse a slight degree of astonishment in my patient. Her surprise manifested itself in the following session. Thoroughly enlivened by a new momentum, my patient stated that, for the first time, she had experienced a very real sense of relief and she continued to be astonished by it. Her usual anxiety had dissipated and she had been able to prepare and give her course calmly, without restlessness and even with pleasure. For her, it was clear that it was the effect of my incongruous remark, and she added that my words "had come from elsewhere and had, as it were, been uttered by an other (*un autre*)"; an other who, she was well aware, was impossible to localise and whose identity was inconceivable. This other, consequently, had just conferred new power on the interpretations that I had provided in vain up until that day. My patient insisted on what had happened. She did not know which was greater: her satisfaction or her astonishment. I shall not speak of my own.

One can easily imagine the discussions and controversies that can be provoked by such an episode. There is matter here for all sorts of theoretical constructions or doctrinal reveries; it even crossed my mind that a comparison could be drawn with the commentary provided by the "*ancient chorus*"!* All this undoubtedly deserves closer examination, but

I will only focus here on what is relevant to my main argument, in other words what forces itself from the outset on our reflections, namely, the identity of this other, who was so talkative. In short, while, on the one hand, it is different from the transference object, on the other I do not think that there is any justification for confusing it with some agency or other that is totally alien to the figures that have left their mark on the history of the subject. I will therefore leave to one side today those aspects that have to do with the identity of my famous "other" in order to focus on one event only, the unexpected emergence of an act of speech whose content was essentially different from what, in other respects, followed its course. My intervention, "And yet, it should have worked!" had the value of an interpretation, even if it did not condemn anything and cannot be entirely explained by what happens in the unconscious. I see my intervention as the ultimate manifestation of a process in the descriptive unconscious, but one that only partly belongs to the systemic unconscious. The process of selecting this and eliminating that had been going on for a long time in my own mind as well as in my patient's, where different words were expected that might permit these interpretations which belonged to the past of the analysis, without having been full cathected, to be integrated and accepted.

It is now possible to return to the hypothesis which seemed to me worthy of attention when I was faced with the questions raised by certain particularities of interpretation.

It is my contention that a special mechanism, of a general order, participates actively and no doubt decisively throughout an analysis in the development of the interpretive process and in the "choice" itself of each of interpretation. But, as I have just pointed out, this mechanism must not be confused with our "instruments" for understanding unconscious scenarios, their evolution and their meaning; it is of another nature. The revelation of unconscious desire and the discovery and analysis of resistance are *functions* of interpretation. Here it is a matter of the *properties* of interpretation,* *which is different*. I will recall them briefly: interpretation is endowed with an evolving structure; it is affected by a certain contingency, since chance plays a part in its emergence; it is actively intolerant, even though, in a form that is often original, it consists, certainly, in suggesting a meaning, but above all in refusing this or that other meaning; it is fruitful because it can give rise to new interpretations or discover itself in other forms; it can behave as a parasite to the point, as we have seen, of producing a separate entity in the analyst's mind and of speaking in his or her place; like an idea, it is apt to progress; it helps the analysand to face up, often successfully, to the dangerous upheavals provoked by the analytic situation; in addition, it protects the analyst, who is also exposed to the risk of psychic disturbance and who is sometimes led to speak and interpret, possibly advisedly, but chiefly to check the deterioration of a regression, to prevent a state of annihilation from establishing itself, or to overcome a state of anarchy in his or her thoughts.

When we reconsider all these properties organically integrated within the interpretation and ready to organise themselves differently in order to engender other interpretations, we see that they are the very properties that characterise *living substance*. In other words, an interpretation, with its remarkable faculty for adapting to the most diverse and dangerous situations, behaves like a *living creature*. Whether it is incisive or incitative, I am ready to attribute it, just like the dream, with a sexual identity! Under these conditions, it is legitimate to suggest that the functioning of interpretation is subject to the decisive activity of the mechanism that governs the fate of living matter, that is to say Darwinian selection* (see *Interpretive Darwinism*). The latter is put in the service of the analyst's instruments of thought, without however undermining the laws of psychic life that our science has established.

Here we are on the frontiers of psychoanalysis, neuroscience and biology. I do not think a priori that there is anything shocking in arguing, as Marc Jeannerod does, that "mental activity, with all its singularity, [has its place] within the general framework of the evolution of biological forms" (Hochmann & Jeannerod, 1991, p. 175); provided, however, and I would like to insist on this point, that thought activities conserve their autonomy, even when they depend fundamentally on the principles that organise life. In any case, by venturing into these regions that separate or link the psychic and the non-psychic, the psychoanalyst is exposed to backing up reflections with an excess of references to disciplines that are incompatible with psychoanalytic doctrine. It will be recalled that in the exchange of letters between Jacques Hochmann and the neurophysiologist Marc Jeannerod, it ultimately emerged that the dissimilar character of their respective lines of research did not allow for a synthesis, even though the dialogue was fascinating and enriching for both domains. As far as I am concerned, I remain sensitive to a remark by Claude Allegre in his *Introduction à une histoire naturelle*:

> Without wishing to philosophize and extend biological lines of reasoning beyond the frontiers within which science seeks to keep them, it might be productive to transpose this kind of reasoning to the domain of the human sciences: culture, languages or populations. Are their respective evolutions not ultimately the result of periods of differentiation and periods of mixing?
>
> (Allègre, 1992, p. 1992, translated for this edition)

Allowing for a mechanism of selection of a Darwinian type in the construction and evolution of interpretation* is nonetheless surprising and requires solid and multiple arguments. Darwin's role in Freud's thought is well known. Lucille Ritvo (1992), who does not overlook the contributions of Jones, Nunberg and Rappaport, has devoted important studies to the subject. She recalls that Freud, on emigrating to London, took with him nine books by Darwin, and that we can find distributed throughout his work, from his *Studies on Hysteria* (1895d) to *Moses and Monotheism* (1939), more than twenty direct references to the illustrious scientist. The Darwinian idea has in short a natural place in Freud's theory of the primal horde or in his thoughts on war. The same cannot be said for a specific psychic activity emerging from mental functioning itself. In "Analysis Terminable and Interminable", Freud (1937a) declines to recognise any other basis for repression than a psychological one. At the very end of the same text, he also argues with regard to penis envy and the repudiation of femininity that if analysis enables us to penetrate the psychological strata of the phenomenon, it ultimately comes up against the famous *bedrock*, a biological obstacle as it were. And Freud adds that, having arrived at this point, "our activities [as analysts] are at an end" (p. 252). In the strict analyst/analysand setting, we are ready to accept that our understanding, at one moment or another, may come up against an insurmountable and fundamental obstacle – is my patient not an illustration of this? – and that it is necessary to lay down one's arms. But when it is a matter of reflecting on our work, which necessarily takes on a speculative character, we cannot recognise any limitations, especially as the task engaged continues to throw up new facts and arguments that legitimise our undertaking. I thus hoped to see the Darwinian thesis of interpretation supported by an examination of the relations between interpretation and construction of the past, two psychic activities in which the activity of memory places a central role.

Today, as in the past, to interpret is to recall. The present of the interpretation is rooted in the past of the analysis, in the past of the analysand and of the analyst alike. By speaking the analyst accepts a historical perspective, but a very particular one because the analyst proposes new versions of what has happened in the analysis and in the patient's history. These new versions do not cancel out the previous ones; rather they are nourished by them and extend them. The patient does not proceed any differently with experienced events, thoughts that he or she has had and the fantasies that he or she has produced, often mixing them all up and turning their chronology upside down. This has the paradoxical advantage, however, of being unifying, of effacing certain discontinuities, of permitting reorganisations and of bringing something new. The interpretative chain, seen from this angle, develops in exactly the same way as the past elaborated on the model of the functioning of memory; in this sense, I agree with André Green (1990a) when he writes that "memory, which by nature is associative, is not only a rediscovery, but a creation . . . thanks to the unceasing transformative power of the mind" (p. 947, translated for this edition). Rediscovery should be understood here in its literal sense, because creation is not spontaneous generation. What was, only exists by being put into the present and reinvented in another form.

Given that the functional similarity between interpretation, construction of the past and memory has been established, am I not justified in thinking that it proceeds from a mechanism that is common to the three activities? This is probably the mechanism whose decisive role appeared to me earlier when I was considering interpretation from the angle of its *properties*. My present starting point is that of *memory*. I found myself particularly interested in this perspective when I discovered the relations between the thesis on the notion of the past that I developed in 1974 in the *International Review of Psychoanalysis* (de M'Uzan, 1974c), which was recently recalled in the *Revue française de psychanalyse* (de M'Uzan, 1988), and the work of Gerald Edelman (1978), as presented by Israël Rosenfeld in 1988, who points out that the views of the biologist specialising in neuroscience are not fundamentally opposed here to the positions of Freud, for whom inexactness in the evocation of memories is a fact. The originality of this work, which I shall review briefly, consists in the fact that it applies a Darwinian theory of the nervous system to the functioning of memory. Neural Darwinism* (see *Interpretive Darwinism*) is now a widely known theory, and holds that the recourse to a principle of natural selection makes it possible to understand partly how perception is organised in relation to the categories that form the basis of memory and recognition. According to this theory, Rosenfeld writes, "each person is unique: his or her perceptions are to some degree creations, and memories are part of an ongoing process of imagination" (1988, p. 193). It may be objected that the focus of interest is purely the formation of perceptual categories and that the question of the higher mental functions is not considered at all. It should be added, however, that, due to their natural upgradeability, these can be included in this way of seeing things. And Rosenfeld, committing himself heavily (but it is very tempting to do so) argues that one can, at the very least, get an intuitive "sense what the biological foundations of mental life might be" (1988, p. 194). I would not go as far as that, of course. But now that I have recalled these considerations, I am in a better position to return to the relations between my view of the role of memory in the edification of the past – and of interpretation which is based on the same model – and that put forward by Israël Rosenfeld, following Gerald Edelman.

In doing so, I am led to recall a number of points of view that will no doubt be familiar to the reader but which are necessary to my line of argument.

The past,* I said at the time, in 1974, is not to be considered as the sum of events of all kinds, deposited in a file storage, sheltered from the wear and tear of time.

For Rosenfeld, our faculty of memorisation is not related to the specific evocation of an image stored somewhere in our brain; in other words, there is no immutable repertoire.

For my part, I saw in the past the rewriting, several times over, of earlier realities reorganised in relation to the situation of the moment, whether of an instinctual drive order, a fantasy-based order, or linked to the environment. The present is the object of a permanent investigation (*instruction*), in the quasi-legal sense of the term, transforming it tendentiously into the past, a past that in turn will be commemorated and betrayed. It is exactly the same with interpretation.

Rosenfeld speaks of an aptitude for organising the surrounding world (that is to say, the present) into general or specific categories, while the needs and desires of the subject determine his way of classifying places, events and individuals. Reorganising and creating is specific to human intelligence. As for memory, its task is not to recall faithfully images and events but to produce new categories. According to the formulation I employed, the old in its initial form is annihilated in favour of a tendentious fable, and the complex exchanges that are established under these circumstances impose a corresponding form on interpretation, as well as the edification of the past, by using selection and introducing variations.

Up to what point is the analyst permitted to follow the neurophysiologist who ventures into the domain of the life of the mind? I do not really know but I stick to a rule whereby, when faced with "something new" and disconcerting, it is initially wise to provisionally suspend all criticism and even to accompany what is proposed in order not to lose anything of it. Since discussion of it only comes afterwards, I felt it was heuristically necessary to take as far as I possibly could the hypothesis of an "*interpretive Darwinism*".* This seems to me to be all the more legitimate in that the selected post of observation is always located in the mental sphere, but *upstream* in relation to our analytic instruments of understanding and interpretation, at the moment when the interpretative "doing" in the sense of the doctrines of phenomenology and poietics is established. In this paper, I have adopted two perspectives that are apparently far removed from each other: that of examining the properties of interpretation, and that of evaluating the role of memory in the fate of interpretations. In each case I have been led to recognise the similar intervention of a mechanism of selection of a Darwinian kind. On the one hand, I discovered in interpretation the characteristics of a living being – gendered, even – and thus subject to the evolutive principle; and, on the other, this same interpretation could be seen developing itself in keeping with the model put forward by neuronal Darwinism, as conceived by Gerard Edelman. A way of thinking, a construction or a hypothesis is more assured, is it not, when reflections of a different nature corroborate it, each from its own angle? Undoubtedly, and this is what I have attempted to do, knowing only too well how problematic a procedure can be that combines two lines of reasoning, one situated in the metaphorical order and the other in the experimental register. In so doing, I am adopting the methods of certain American researchers such as C.F.A. Pantin, when he posits, following R.A. Hinde (1960), that

> The models in biology are all the more promising . . . in that they are sufficiently concrete to be related to the types of mechanism which, at a given stage of the science concerned, are capable of being studied in organisms while at the same time sufficiently abstract to reveal new possibilities and new quantitative relationships.
>
> (Pantin, 1968, pp. 194–195)

I therefore considered that the notion of "interpretative Darwinism"* was sufficiently well founded and that consequently some of its theoretical implications could be considered. The essential ones are the notion of functional continuity, which includes the question of memory traces; the problem of the discharge of excitation; and, finally, the place of perception.* I can do no more than sketch their outlines here.

It is clear that the Darwinian thesis contains the idea of a continuity between biological neuronal and psychic processes, which in no way excludes leaps and mutations. But given the heterogeneity of these three orders, and especially the last two, the continuity in question can only be functional; in other words, the result of a permanent activity which only the work of a selective mechanism operating both at the neuronal level and at the level of the life of the mind can help us understand. The arguments interact and are mutually supportive. There is no fixed state of life, except mineral, and even then . . . ! Billions of neurons and tens of billions of synapses can only be conceived, therefore, as being constantly at work, involved in a continual activity which, were it to stop for a single moment, would bring about a change of order in the structures concerned. Michel Jouvet (1992, p. 126) says that this continuity subsists even in deep sleep. He points out that this idea is not a new one by citing the pithy remark made by the theologian Ralph Cudworth to René Descartes in 1678: "The sleeping geometer never ceases in a certain way to have within himself all his geometrical theorems, just as the sleeping musician also conserves all his musical aptitudes and his melodies" (ibid., p. 126, translated for this edition); and I would add, especially since they have not ceased for a single moment to repeat them to themselves, at the heart of the most impenetrable regions of their mind.

The same is true of the construction of the past, of the psychic processes that lead to interpretation and, undoubtedly, of mental life as a whole.

Perceiving, repeating, selecting: we only recall what we have not ceased for a single moment to tell ourselves in the form of a *deep narrative* which duplicates, as if in counterpoint, both waking life and that which proceeds from unconscious impulses and from the activity of their representations in fantasies and dreams. Interpretative activity, with all its richness, depends fundamentally on this incessant work carried out beneath or beyond the systemic Unconscious, without the analyst knowing it. I conceive it as endless kind of *rumination* or rambling, so to speak, which begins in the first moments of the first session and takes shape thanks to a differential selection into which our unconscious processes, in the precise sense of the term, only enter partially. This shaping does not concern static states of fixed representations, but modes of functioning which I would readily call *deep memory*. In the armchair, analysts are not faced with a series of paintings hanging on the wall of their conscious awareness. They discern emergences – in the quasi biological sense of the term – of what they have more or less vaguely heard in their patients' utterances; emergences that silently continue to develop at a distance from their consciousness before culminating, in the light of day, in a formulated interpretation. This being the case, it is probable that all that can be selected is what at the beginning, and even during the briefest unit of time, had benefited from a sufficient libidinal cathexis. Failing which, the event will not be the object of a *true forgetting*, that is to say symptomatic, but will have been excluded from the recitative fabric owing to the activation of a selective mechanism; and it is not recoverable. It is amnesia. Amnesia is not forgetting, as André Green (1990b, p. 182) has pointed out. And the amnesia of which he speaks owes nothing to repression which, in fact, protects memory. What cannot in any case be recalled and represented thanks to the lifting of repression is what, independently of the lack of libidinal cathexis referred to earlier, has often been the victim of a brutal event, of an economic order, and consequently put out of play. This can be observed especially in so-called "psychosomatic" structures.

Thus, two narratives at least will unfold in front of the analyst. The first, which we are familiar with, proceeds from the vicissitudes of unconscious processes; the second, which permits and serves the first, organises the web of perceptions by recalling them and transforming them infinitely. In speaking of an event of an economic order, capable of impeding the edification of the deep narrative or of shattering its development, I was thinking, among other things, of an extreme act: the discharge of cathexes. Discharge makes it possible, certainly, to eliminate what has not been accepted or legitimised. But more often than not *discharge is the misfortune of memory*. André Green admits as much by saying that the mind is only controllable because it is no longer automatically discharged (ibid., p. 194). I think, therefore, that it is indeed due to a selective action that the energy involved in a perception* can either be discharged or cathected, taking up again indefinitely what has just happened, and thereby become the object of new perceptions.

The evolutive point of view concerning psychic facts, in particular, memory storage and interpretation, leads to many theoretical reorganisations. Thus the idea that Freud held for a time that psychic processes correspond to quantitatively determined states of material particles can no longer be admitted.

To do so, it would be necessary for static, fixed registrations to exist, but this runs contrary to living substance which does not tolerate the slightest immobility in what serves as a support for images. Strictly speaking, then, one cannot speak of memory traces; for it is not fixed images that are perceived, but the destiny of continuous series of perceptions organised into categories in order to constitute the basis of a narrative. Is this not what André Green means when he writes: "Meaning takes precedence over the simplifying vision of the recollection of memories . . . [and] memory is based in fact on a phenomenon of perceptual anticipation" (ibid.)?

I now want to say a brief word concerning the last of the three theoretical implications mentioned above.

As we progress in our examination of the various phenomena in which the task of memory is involved, we discover at each step the decisive role of perception,* which is really an activity of selection. It is well known that we learn not by retaining but by eliminating. The psychical apparatus continually perceives everything that is derived from the internal world and from the external world so that "what is seen" becomes the object of an incessant and increasingly complex perceptual and selective activity, thereby constituting, for a large part, the psychic domain. It would be tempting to see what the outcome would be of a reflection on the functioning of the mind that took perception as a central reference, something Freud, at the time of the "Project" (1950)[1895]) had imagined up to a certain point.

Now that I have reached the end of my statement, and since its impact on our ordinary practice is not immediately evident, it may be asked why, on the subject of interpretation, I have ventured into this area situated between the neuronal and the mental. An abyss for some, a barrier for others, the alternative is laden with philosophical consequences. For my part, I would like to see only a transitional area, thereby exposing myself to Freud's friendly reproach of Groddeck for quietly mixing the psychic and the somatic and doing away with "beautiful differences" (Letter of 5 June 1917, in E.L. Freud, 1960, p. 324). And what if, in choosing my subject, I may have been influenced by some obscure Darwinian mechanism? Unless, having been absorbed so often and at such length by the question of interpretation, I found myself in the situation described by a Tamil proverb that often comes to my mind and that Jean Paulhan sometimes used in his dedications: "When one is sitting on a tiger, one cannot stop when one wants to".

Note

1 This chapter was first published as an article in the *Revue française de psychanalyse*, 57 (1): 7–20 in 1993.

Part III

Glossary of the main notions

Elaborated by the author

MURIELLE GAGNEBIN

Architecture and continuity in Michel Émile de M'Uzan's thought

This glossary[1] should make it possible to follow the evolution of a way of thinking that has the potential to reform many aspects of psychoanalysis and to open up new paths of thinking concerning the act of analysis, on the one hand, and the forms of analytic treatment on the other.

For many years a fervent advocate of the purest form of drive functioning as the eminent locus of psychoanalysis, tracking it down to the point of turning the analytic session into an erogenous zone – a sort of living creature possessing a precise psychic structure like an individual and a destiny like a person, and even endowing interpretation with a sexual identity – de M'Uzan rejects both the "orthopaedic" theories of *Ego Psychology* of the Hartmannian type and deviations that quite simply do away with *affect* or, at the other extreme, promote "holding" techniques worthy of the children's playground.

De M'Uzan acquired clinical experience over more than twenty years of the heavy psychosomatic situations one is faced with in hospitals (haemorrhagic rectocolitis, Crohn's disease, widespread eczema, severe asthma, giant psoriasis, lung diseases, etc.), and understood that alongside the importance of instinctual drive functioning, an important place had to be reserved for failures in questions of identity (*l'identitaire*) which he was to place within an order where what he calls the *"vital-identital"** reigns, and where very serious and lethal progressions sometimes take place. This is why he was led to conceive two orders, one geared towards narcissistic and object-related drive functioning, the other towards vacillations of identity, the abysses of depersonalisations* even leading to the exhaustion of being, where the sexual, castration and mentalisation no longer obtain. This led him to add to the strictly libidinal epistemology the necessity of listening to a continuous bass which he called the *programme of life with death at the end*, where the *vital-identital* is operative. Consequently, in analytic work it is a matter of being closely involved in the *negotiations** between these two orders, negotiations that involve an intense use of the *perceptual dimension*. This implied inventing a new grammar specific to interventions-interpretations, a grammar drawing on the most disturbing and dizzy experiences of depersonalisation and regression, which is a "way" of helping the patient gain access once again to mentalisation via a perceptual closeness involving the analyst's very person. Take, for instance, the extremely depersonalised and fragmented woman patient, who no longer felt anything but a sense of suffocating formlessness, to whom de M'Uzan said calmly, "Your contours are in my pocket" (see Chapter 6, p. 87 THIS TEXT; 2008a, p. 48; 2013b, p. 170), linking in this way the perceptual and libidinal dimensions. De M'Uzan's thought is tirelessly concerned with revealing the entanglements between these two orders.

The aim of this glossary is to introduce the reader to this process and to retrace the adventure of a psychoanalysis which promises not so much "cure" (or cure as an additional benefit, as has been said), but much more a state of *permanent disquiet** as a fundamental economic status of being; or, if one prefers, the passion for an asymptotic perfectibility in the analytic understanding of oneself, which, in an article on the end of analysis, de M'Uzan (1997) called *"Les yeux de Chimène"*. How can one better place oneself deliberately at the heart of what is most *alive* (*vivante*), where the economic and "psychisation" (i.e. inscription in the psychosexual register) prevail, even including the dignity of the process of dying, the individual's ultimate psychic attempt to put him- or herself paradoxically once again in the world! And I would add, to make dying (obviously when the subject can) a final work of art, in the sense of a creative expression of meaning. You may recall the death of the writer Bergotte in Proust. Wanting, in spite of his diminishing strength, to go and contemplate the "little patch of yellow wall" in Vermeer's 1660 painting "View of Delft", the writer suddenly understood that the painter must have superimposed several layers, something he (Bergotte) felt he ought to have done in his own writing. Nourished by this enriching understanding, it was not long before Bergotte collapsed and died.

I have chosen to order this glossary alphabetically, but the chronological references of de M'Uzan's texts, where the notions and their definitions appear for the first time, and are subsequently developed, indicate the maturation of a process of reflection spreading over a life entirely devoted to clinical analysis and metapsychology. It is worth noting that, in his very first writings, de M'Uzan had a sense of what this form of clinical practice would be for him – one that he also advocated in view of the fact that its discoveries have so many repercussions. In this connection, he spoke of *"Reconsidérations et nouveaux développements en psychanalyse"* (see de M'Uzan, 2011b; 2013b, pp. 187–200). This is why I would prefer to speak of an evolution and enrichment of his thought rather than of ruptures and contradictions. What emerged in a veiled form right at the beginning follows an increasingly precise and ever deeper trajectory which culminates in introducing into the Freudian and post-Freudian hermeneutics paths, which, albeit totally innovative, it is true, are ones that Freud would surely not have disavowed. Indeed, respect for the Freudian "thing" is maintained from one end to the other, including in the extensions and blossomings furnished by de M'Uzan, which were only possible thanks to intransigent reflection on his own clinical practice. His thoroughly unique and ingenious creativity, quite apart from the highly unusual directions and methods that it resulted in, remain a tribute to the father of psychoanalysis.

Actings

Direct *acting out* represents a discharge that does not take up an element of the *written past* as is the case in the *actings* linked to the "transference neurosis".* *Acting out* is not the equivalent of a recollection, but rather the trace of an action that probably had the same mechanical appearance. Conceived as the repetition of a repetition, it can assume the significance of a scream that does not enter into a construction implying the presence of a third party. As a qualitative degradation of energy, it seems to obey the principle of nirvana alone and is often the mark of an organic illness.

Acting in is the equivalent of a somatic symptom indicating what is being played out in the order of the *"vital-identital"*.* (See "Acting Out 'Direct' et Acting Out 'Indirect'" [1967, 1977, pp. 75–82]; see also "The Slaves of Quantity" [1984]. See also *Vital-identital* in this glossary.)

Actual psychosis

Under this term, de M'Uzan places nosographical entities whose formation is derived neither from a work of the ego bearing on instinctual drive representations, nor from a confrontation with a return of the repressed within the context of *représentance*. Thus, alongside the "actual neuroses" defined by Freud, the author has identified the "actual psychoses" involved in the constitution of somatoses. These psychoses, which de M'Uzan calls "actual", are thus non-delusional. Consequently, they attest to a deficiency of mentalisation and a loss of cathectic energy. It is worth noting here that for de M'Uzan there are "two points of entry into psychosis", as he writes himself when he refers to his "red line or line of meaning",* "from above" (for the delusional psychoses) and "from below" (for the actual psychoses, those pertaining to the *"vital-identital"**); drama, on the one hand, and tragedy on the other, he adds. (See de M'Uzan, 2011g, pp. 17–23.)

In order to grasp clearly what de M'Uzan means by "actual psychoses", it is necessary to take stock of some closely related yet very different notions that tend to be amalgamated.

For André Green and Jean-Luc Donnet, "blank psychosis" ("*psychose blanche*") affects thought itself insofar as the subject feels he or she has gone blank, is incapable of thinking, feels empty, or that he or she has holes in the head. This blank represents an absence of representations. "Blank psychosis" for these authors functions like a paralysis of thought and is linked to the concept of the "dead mother" (Green, 1980), a mother who is indifferent to her newborn baby, depressive, preoccupied by other concerns: mourning, abandonment, etc., and with the concept of "negative hallucination", which, for Green, it should be recalled, is the precondition for positive hallucination. The subject uses negative hallucination because he prefers to avoid seeing himself at all, rather than seeing himself suffering and degraded (see Green & Donnet, 1973; Green, 1983).

For Évelyne Kestemberg, on the other hand, "cold psychosis" is a defensive mode aimed at resolving anxiety, primary, vital and unbearable anxiety, which makes the clinician working with such patients experience a sense of vacuity. It is a psychosis without delusion and it is the "inanimate" dimension of the object that gives this kind of psychosis, in which the subject has fallen back on forms of auto-erotism, its "cold" colour. The concept of "cold psychosis" is to be seen in relation to the concept of the "fetishist relationship to the object" worked out by É. Kestemberg, a transference/countertransference indicator of this organisation (see Kestemberg, 2001).

As can be seen, the question presents itself quite differently for de M'Uzan.

For him, "actual psychosis" is very close to the psychosomatic concept of "operational thinking" (*pensée opératoire*). It is a defence against the consequences of a psychic defence, foreclosure or "*Verwerfung*". "Actual psychosis" is dementalised, drive functioning has no place in it; we are deep inside the "*vital-identital*".* De M'Uzan is thus led to dismember the notion of "actual energy". The "actual neuroses" (anxiety neurosis, essential depression, psychosomatic breakdown, etc.) are classically opposed to the psychoneuroses, first and foremost, anxiety hysteria. They are driven by "an energy 'without quality' proceeding from a loss of quality of the libido". However, there is still

> an *actual energy*, also without quality, unrelated to the libido, but non-pathological and in the service of self-preservation; that is, in the service of different organic functions (cerebral included) both at the level of their activity and of their period of existence.
>
> (de M'Uzan, 2005a, p. 122, translated for this edition)

This is what leads, for de M'Uzan, to the constitution of a "flagstone of identity",* that is, to an irresistible formation at the heart of "organic being" (see *"das organische Wesen"* according to Freud (1991) (*Gesammelte Werke*, XIV, pp. 119–120). De M'Uzan adds:

> Just as libidinal energy can lose its quality, the actual energy of self-preservation can, for its part, become degraded and lapse into anarchic modes of functioning, as can be observed in some of the most serious somatoses, in respect of which I have spoken or *actual psychoses*.
>
> (2005a, p. 122)

On the one hand, then, there are the "actual neuroses" under the sway of a quantitative factor capable of compelling "a libido that has become wild first to regress and to express itself in the perverse mode; and then, as the process continues, to lose its qualities so that it is no longer anything but pure energy of excitation" (ibid.). On the other, there are the "actual neuroses" which are also governed by the quantitative. De M'Uzan continues:

> The same is true of the actual energy of self-preservation when it is subject to the tyranny of quantity and is no longer capable of serving an integrated physiological functioning. The shadow of the principle of inertia, an agent of stasis or of total discharge is then cast.
>
> (ibid.)

(See "À l'Horizon. Le facteur actuel" [2001]; see also "Reconsiderations and New Developments in Psychoanalysis" [2011b]).

Aim of analysis

For de M'Uzan it is above all a matter of helping the patient to enlarge his or her mental functioning and to achieve a *psychic mutation*. You will recall the woman patient who told him: "I would like to have a good hammer to be able smash your skull and to see what is inside". "To be more exact", de M'Uzan continues, "the interest that she showed for the contents of my mind, among which she was supposed to occupy a prominent position, masked an obscure curiosity about my mental functioning" (see "During the Session" [1989]).

For Freud, analytic treatment was above all *about working on conscious and unconscious representations* in the hope of promoting a process of *rebinding* at the heart of the psychical apparatus. For de M'Uzan, the analytic motor is not to be sought first and foremost in the activity or movement of representation (*représentance*) (as in J. Lacan, W.R. Bion, A. Green, etc.), but rather in a *seism* affecting these same so-called secondary systems. In his view, only a preliminary task, aimed principally, and in a new way, at shaking up the quietude of the ego, at provoking an economic scandal, is likely to liberate the energy necessary for an original cathexis. For him, it is thus a matter of placing oneself at the very heart of *unbinding*, favouring moments of depersonalisation in analysand and analyst alike, permitting the creation of what he has called the *chimera*. (See "The Mouth of the Unconscious" [1978a; this volume]; see also *Psychological chimera* and *Depersonalisation* in this glossary.)

Subsequently, de M'Uzan was to add yet another function: the analyst must introduce at the end of the analysis a state of "permanent disquiet"* in the analysand which will push him or her to engage in self-analysis or to do successive analyses. (See "Invitation to Frequent the Shadows" [2006]).

Analytic grammar

Like K.A. Kemper (1965) and analysts in France who counted for him in various respects (S. Nacht, M. Bouvet), de M'Uzan advocates "brief, incomplete and ambiguous" interventions designed to leave "the patient an almost creative freedom" because they do not hinder the "tendency towards discovery". Contrary to the interpretation-explanation that always resonates, more or less, like a conclusion strongly tinged by the colours of the analyst, de M'Uzan forges an "original grammar" structured like jokes, dreams or symptoms, which is therefore able to convince the preconscious of the patient. By basing his interventions on certain primary processes such as displacement and especially condensation, he avoids in the first place the trap of interpretation-intrusion; next, he short-circuits several defences and, in keeping with the aim of analysis, gives the patient the possibility of bringing about a certain *psychic mutation*. At this precise moment, and only at this moment, since the economic dimension has been briefly disturbed, the analysand has the opportunity of undergoing a *psychic reorganisation* (see de M'Uzan [1983b]). However, having distinguished two orders of functioning, those of drive activity and the "*vital-identital*",* de M'Uzan, far from giving up his initial interpretations, adds, during the *negotiations** that he carries out between these two orders with a view to bringing the patient back into the axis of the libidinal sphere, interpretations that are based above all on *perceptual activity*. The originality of his grammar is thereby all the greater. (See "De l'informe avant toute chose", 2003a.)

Ancient chorus

For de M'Uzan, in the exchange between the analysand and the analyst, the statements of the protagonists do not always belong to the psychosexual order. At these moments, ideally the analyst should not speak in the first person, with in addition the identity of "armchair giant" (Lacan).

He should speak using the impersonal pronoun "one", which de M'Uzan calls the "ancient chorus", in order to participate in the famous "flagstone of identity".* "This in no way prevents one from setting up the conditions that are necessary to ensure, when the time comes, the place of the sexual in the transference" (see "Réponse à Clarisse Baruch", 2011c).

Arborescent activity

Employing a vegetal metaphor, de M'Uzan recommends "arborescent activity" in the analysand. The associations will therefore be marked as much by the gap that disunites them as by the lasting nature of a link that connects them at the starting point of the sequence, affirming an undeniable continuity. It is a very particular dynamic in which one can recognise the characteristic growth of a tree. For de M'Uzan this arborescent activity characterises the optimal functioning of free association; the author is led to substitute the idea of change for the ideal of cure. Furthermore, this functioning, when it occurs easily, is also one of the signs of the end of analysis. (See "Du derangement au changement" [1991, 1994b, p. 126].)

Basic tonus of identity

Of genetic origin, it emanates from the programme of creation, development and preservation of the human being. If it is in deficit, the subject will try to obtain it from a toxic source (heroin, cocaine, various drugs). In adulthood, subjects whose tonus of identity is deficient are plunged into a determining situation of economic and quantitative debt. Because the forces of self-preservation are affected, the drug addict is a "slave of quantity" by default. (See "The Slaves of quantity" [1984].)

Castration anxiety

Usually castration anxiety is experienced by a boy as the fulfilment of a paternal threat in response to his sexual activities. In a girl, the absence of a penis is experienced as a loss incurred that she tries to deny, compensate or repair.

For de M'Uzan, the question is posed quite differently.

First, he shows that bulbocavernous erectile bodies are identical in men and women, except that they are *reunited and externalised* in the penis for men, whereas, for women, both cavernous bodies are *internal*, located in the pelvic floor, on both sides of the vaginal walls. The first conclusion is that irrespective of the experience that accompanies it, the phenomenon of orgasm is consequently basically *identical* for both sexes. It is *one* and must be distinguished both from jouissance, from pleasure and from the capacity for erogeneity that characterises almost the entire human body, including the vaginal walls and even – the surgical consequence of a colon pathology – the mouth of an artificial anus.

Second, he draws attention to one of the most poignant misunderstandings for a woman. As the victim of an imaginary castration, is she not led to exhibit herself sometimes *entirely* as a penis, that is, like an erectile body that she does not know she possesses already, albeit *within* herself? And de M'Uzan cites the irresistible fluorescent blue sheath dresses in the manner of San Antonio or the one-piece, black leather suits clinging to undulating waists, topped by long shimmering and twirling hair, in the style of Pieyre de Mandiargues. Metonymy is thus all the rage and similar affirmations bring with them a procession of psychic mutilations and painful social aberrations.

Finally, and this is undoubtedly the most interesting point for de M'Uzan, the question of castration is considered "as a chance for the human imagination" (1964, 1977, p. 8) insofar as it develops the "integrative capacities of the individual". Considered henceforth as phallic, the libido, one and indivisible, is combined with a biological and physiological tendency towards *integration* (Gagnebin, 1996, p. 50). Once again, de M'Uzan speaks in favour of a maturational value conducive to the creative process, and entirely to the glory of the inventive human spirit. (See the minutes of the seminar given at the Institute of Psychoanalysis of the Paris Psychoanalytic Society in 1994–1995, titled "Conséquences psychologiques des différences et des similitudes anatomiques de la femme et de l'homme"; and particularly "Aperçus sur le processus de la creation littéraire" [1964]; see also *De l'art à la mort*, 1977a, p. 8.)

Death drive

De M'Uzan rejects the existence of the death drive, and subscribes to Jones's thesis that in 1915 we already had a complete edifice of Freudian metapsychology. The death drive thus appears as a sort of conceptual aberration, for the individual does not explode but rather implodes, or better, dies. We speak of the "last breath". Furthermore, what would the somatic source of this death drive be?

De M'Uzan prefers to speak of a *special fate of the instinct*, whose ultimate term is not an active destruction – division, fragmentation – but a veritable *extinction*. He also separates the death instinct from destructive forces. A destructive process is something that is the cause of divisions, splits and perhaps disorganisations. But clinical experience shows that, at the level of fantasy, life can perfectly well continue in each of the parts that result from the fragmentation. Moreover, he recognises that there are phenomena for which the idea of a lethal tendency seems to impose itself: repetition of the same, traumatic neuroses, negative therapeutic reaction, etc. The "actual" factor then dominates and a tendency towards total extinction of the excitation can be observed. These kinds of process involving such a fatal outcome have been seen as the effects of a special instinct. De M'Uzan has opted therefore for a *special fate of the instinct*. Profoundly monistic (only the libidinal drive exists), he envisages a dualism of differentiation or of destiny. (See de M'Uzan, 1972; 1977, pp. 125–150; 1963; 2015.) De M'Uzan thus remains in the continuity of Freud who, in 1925, and therefore at a late stage in his work, wrote:

> But the unconscious seems to contain nothing that could give any content to our concept of the annihilation of life. . . . I am therefore inclined to adhere to the view that the fear of death should be regarded as analogous to the fear of castration.
>
> (Freud, 1926, pp. 129–130)

This text signifies for de M'Uzan, without any shadow of doubt, "the death of death" (see de M'Uzan, 1968; 1977, p. 52). In the systemic unconscious, there is no place for this concept. Jones highlights this point, speaking of the Freud of 1915: "Had his work come to an end then, we should have possessed a well-rounded account of psychoanalysis in what might be called its classical form" (Jones, 1957, p. 265). Freud always recognised the existence of destructive tendencies which he linked initially to the ego-instincts, which work with them for the survival of the individual (otherwise humankind would still have webbed fingers!), and then to the libido with which they collude in perverse behaviours. In short, for de M'Uzan, and from a perfectly classical Freudian standpoint, there is no death drive in the unconscious. *Destrudo* is first and foremost a *principle of functioning* that features in the genetic programme of the individual, a programme of life, of duration of life; secondly, *destrudo* (so violent and obvious in wars, the ferocious taste for extermination and genocides that ravaged the 20th century and continue in the 21st) pertains to a perversion of the cultural order but certainly not of a *death drive* inherent in the human mind: once again, the systemic unconscious only knows what is analogous to it, namely, castration. (See "The Corrida . . . and Its Nether Side" [2011; this volume]; and "Réponse à Sylvie Faure-Pragier" [2011f]).

It is worth recalling, once again, that for de M'Uzan dying is a work that enables the individual (when he or she can) to complete the instinctual drive integration and thus to pursue self-creation. (See *Work of dying* in this glossary.)

Depersonalisation

To this concept studied by Maurice Bouvet (1960), de M'Uzan adds that phenomena of depersonalisation can occur without being accompanied by anxiety, but rather by a certain exaltation, as can be observed during so-called creative activities or sports exercises that have been "completely mastered". It is as if the "activity of perception" had supplanted every other activity or function (see "Intervention by de M'Uzan" in Rome at the 21st Congress of French-Speaking Psychoanalysts on the Report by Maurice Bouvet [1960] "Dépersonnalisation et relations d'objet", *RFP*, 24, pp. 4–5, pp. 630–634). That being so, de M'Uzan was to speak throughout his work of *distressing* phenomena of depersonalisation which could also serve as the lever for creation, both in analysis and in art. For him, as for Bouvet, depersonalisation is related to a disturbance of the psychic economy. The subject no longer recognises him- or herself, contours become blurred, the head seems to empty itself or to be invaded by strange ideas or images: it is as if the subject's identity were disappearing. When these phenomena are slight, they announce the emergence of the *chimera,** without which, for de M'Uzan, "there is no true analysis", and are closely related to what he calls the "paradoxical system".* They have their roots in the loose soil of uncanniness. When the phenomena of depersonalisation are violent, the subject seems to slip out of the libidinal, narcissistic and objected-related order towards the order de M'Uzan calls the *"vital-identital"*.* The risk then arises of falling into what de M'Uzan calls the "actual psychoses"* or even of triggering somatoses. The subject then no longer has access to mentalisation. (See "Affect et processus d'affectation" [1970]; "The Mouth of the Unconscious" [1978a; this volume]; and finally, "The Uncanny or 'I Am Not Who You Think I Am'" [2009].) In *Aux confins de l'identité*, de M'Uzan (2005a) looks extensively at the dark sides of depersonalisation.* (See in particular the chapters "The Paraphrenic Twin or at the Frontiers of Identity" [1999, 2005a, pp. 15–40]; "De l'informe avant toute chose" [2003, 2005a, pp. 100–109]; "Séparation et identité" [2001, 2005a, pp. 124–131]; "Addiction et problématique identitaire: le 'tonus de base'" [2004, 2005a, pp. 132–141]; and "Le développement identitaire: accomplissements et achoppements" [2005a, pp. 142–164].) (See also *Paradoxical system* and *Actual psychosis* in this glossary.)

Difference between the two topographies

Proposing real characters (the id, the ego, the superego), the second topography (1920) is akin, according to de M'Uzan, to a "scenario" which, in order to become manifest, needs a *mise en scène*. Indeed, for him, this is the exact function of the first topography (*Ucs., Pcs. and Cs*). De M'Uzan gives priority, then, to the metapsychology of 1915 insofar as it serves the economic dimension more and leads to a *realisation* whose only scenario, left to itself, seems private, offering itself more perhaps to "textual analysis" and thus to the thrills of conceptual scaffolding. (See the minutes of the seminar given at the Paris Institute of Psychoanalysis [SPP] on the

"Conséquences psychologiques des differences et des similitudes anatomiques de la femme et de l'homme", session of 4 July 1995.)

Drive

For de M'Uzan, the drive is an *invention* of the psychical apparatus which, as Freud claimed, is a *fiction*. (See "A New Perspective in Psychoanalysis" [2008b; this volume].)

Egg-laying, covetousness, domination

These are the three mechanisms that account for the predominance in every analyst of very different unconscious psychic mechanisms – dispositions, moreover, that can vary from patient to patient. Covetousness is thus a feature of the analyst who is greedy with regard to psychic contents identified in the patient; that is to say enthralled by the patient's history and therefore by his or her narratives, and even capable of nourishing on them. Egg-laying is perhaps more characteristic of the Kleinian, always ready to deposit, like an egg, his or her interpretation in the patient's mind. Finally, domination refers to a particular interest in the patient's mental functioning: structures of thought, the sequence of ideas and the ellipses of reasoning are closely tracked with the aim of making sure the analyst is in control of them. The analyst is less interested here in life stories, arising from daily biography, than in their rhetoric, their *mise en scène*. (See "During the Session" [1989].)

Ego of the Ego

For de M'Uzan, "the ego of the Ego" is an agency detached from the ego through *splitting*. It has the task of accepting and fully recognising the strictly mortal character of every living organism. It enables the individual to mourn the self from day to day, whereas someone who *denies death* continues to be active as if he or she were immortal until the end, thanks to the *penetration* of the voice of the Unconscious into all levels of the "psychical apparatus". De M'Uzan writes:

> I would suggest, then, that when the splitting in question has occurred, there is a collusion between self-preservation, even operating in desperation, and the certainty of death. In other words, the "ego of the Ego" plots with self-preservation *behind the back* of the unconscious [which is unaware of death, negation and time] with the aim of reducing its activity as much as possible.
>
> (2013b, p. 122)

The marginalisation of the voice of the unconscious, at a moment when it is important that it can make itself heard, constitutes, in his view, a privation of freedom, a mutilation of the subject. In this sense, Christian David's position, according to which, *mourning for oneself, in advance, is a necessity*, could lend support to the *stoic* position (see David, 1996). De M'Uzan (2013b) continues: "The primordial purpose of the first of these orientations is to carry out stoically a process of mourning for oneself; the aim of the second is to take the self-construction of a human being as far as possible" (p. 134), and he adds,

> for me nothing must be allowed to defeat the instinct which compels every living thing to cling to life (in keeping with Freud's ideas in "Mourning and Melancholia" [1917, p. 246]), that is to say to live psychically, to continue to develop itself to the very limit, without this entailing an alteration of the continuity of object-cathexis.
>
> (de M'Uzan, 2013b, p. 135)

On the one hand there is *philosophical melancholy* and, on the other, the creativity of Socrates-psychoanalyst who, on the eve of his death, obeys a recurring dream telling him: "Make music! Be productive!" This confirms the psychoanalytic experience of de M'Uzan who accompanied his patients up until the last moment and noticed, as death approached, "a libidinal expansion and the exaltation of an appetite for relationships" (2013b, p. 120). (See "Death Never Confesses" [1996]; and also "The Work of Dying" [1976a].)

Energy without quality

The author makes a distinction in many texts between the quantitative and the qualitative. "Slaves of quantity" are subject to a regime governing non-libidinal energy. Their fate depends on pure discharge. They sometimes look for other solutions such as drugs, exploits in sport, etc. The analytic work must allow this energy without quality to transform itself gradually. Energy without quality is the regime of the "vital-identital".* (See "The Slaves of Quantity" [1984].)

Flagstone of identity

De M'Uzan evokes on more than one occasion the fundamental formation of a "flagstone of identity". This *flagstone of identity* concerns the classical theory of "anaclisis". For de M'Uzan, the emergence of the sexual drive is not underpinned by "self-preservation" alone, as it was conceived classically with Freud in 1915, but on what he calls the "vital-identital",* of which self-preservation without its instinctual drive substratum is part.

The "burgeoning" of the erogenous zones proceeds from the initiation of an "essentially genetic programme" that began "with the meeting between male and female gametes, in a sufficiently hazardous way to create a role for history" (see de M'Uzan, 2011c, p. 24; 2013b, p. 193). The execution of this programme of life, with its stages (trauma of birth, differentiation of the archaic self from itself, birth of the paraphrenic twin,* tendentious messages of the mother or of the *Nebenmensch* [of the person who is there to take care of the infant], "maternal" seduction contaminated by her own unconscious, puberty, menopause or andropause, death at the end) and its determined duration, depends first on the engagement of energy which is initially "without quality" and produced essentially by intracellular formations, mitochondria. Thus the history of the development of the being is also one of the destiny of energy, of force, of which the economic point of view will be the metapsychological "echo" when the subject has attained a psychosexual status. There is justification, therefore, for speaking of a certain parallelism between the evolution of "organic being", the *"vital-identital"** or the formation of the "flagstone of identity", in the direction of the "psychosexual subject" and the evolution of the status of an energy that is initially without quality, and in the service of the integrated functioning of the organism, towards libidinal drive activity. Clearly, it is not a matter of substituting one order or status for another, but of various degrees of entanglement. This essentially genetic programme (the *"vital-identital"**) is thus marked by the "seductive message" of the adult, that is, of an other. The temporal gap – even if minimal – between the initiation of the *"vital-identital"* and of the *sexual* (Laplanche, 2007) is inevitable since the latter depends on the seductive intervention of the other. A link is therefore provided between seduction and the problematic of identity. Thus an "evolutive negotiation" is established between these two orders. The extended biological order is also distinguished from the purely physiological order. And, once again, the economic dimension prevails: it is once again a question of a demand for psychic work. (See *Aux confins de l'identité* [2005a]; "Reconsiderations and New Developments in Psychoanalysis" [2011b, pp. 23–24; 2015a, p. 118; 2013b, p. 192].)

Inner public

This is a sort of composite internal image closely linked to the parental couple and which determines the work of creation. De M'Uzan writes:

> The inner public, which is the mediator, the dedicatee and, in a sense, the progenitor of the work, is endowed with a psychic reality which appears for us above all in the disorders it causes as soon as it no longer fulfils exactly all its roles. Indeed, its very existence can easily be the source of unconscious guilt, for it presupposes a withdrawal

> of cathexis from the outer world, which it does away with, at least momentarily; what is more, the new father that one gives oneself in this way implies an elimination of the real father, which, unconsciously, can only be experienced as a murder. The writer must therefore begin by reconciling him or herself with a megalomaniac usurping of power, the first effect of which is a destructive act.
>
> (1964, 1977, p. 21)

De M'Uzan also warns against making a "fusion between the inner public and a maternal image" which would be a fixation full of complications. (See de M'Uzan, 1964; 1977, pp. 3–27.) It is clear that this "inner public", which de M'Uzan sometimes likens to an "inner character", is quite similar to "an *alter ego* of the author who seeks, via this detour, to restore his narcissistic integrity". It should thus not be confused with the notion proposed by Murielle Gagnebin (2011) of *Ego alter*, which, for her, is the emergence, at a certain moment during the initial elaboration of the work, of a force inherent to it which dictates its laws to the artist, and which, in this way, dispossesses him or her momentarily of his or her creation by revealing the *autonomy of the work*. M. Gagnebin's notion of *Ego alter*, which plays a role in the elaboration of the artistic field, is linked in several ways with de M'Uzan's *chimera* when it emerges in the analytic treatment.

For de M'Uzan, if the *chimera* (see *Psychological chimera*),* the fruit of the "spectrum of identity" which validates the "paradoxical system",* does not constitute itself, there is no real analysis; likewise, for M. Gagnebin, the appearance of the *Alter ego* guarantees the authenticity of a work.

Interpretation

Interpretation should be *mutative*. De M'Uzan thus evaluates the chances of success by making interpretation a real *living creature*, following in so doing a sort of "interpretive Darwinism" based on selection (see *Interpretive Darwinism* in this glossary). The danger of an "immune" defence is explored in the process. Interpretation must therefore avoid three temptations: *covetousness* (coveting the contents of the patient's discourse); *egg-laying* (depositing, like eggs in a nest, problems that belong to the analyst); and *domination* (exercising tight control over the links in the patient's discourse).

He also proposes a very special grammar of interpretation favouring the emergence of a disturbance of identity characteristic of a reorganisation of the psychic economy. It may then give the impression of having been offered by an *other* (see *Psychological chimera* in this glossary). In so doing, and employing a military or playful metaphor (chess), de M'Uzan contrasts Freudian conceptions which depend, according to him, on a *strategy*, with Kleinian conceptions which obey the requirements of *tactics*.

In this way he is led to distinguish between three types of past involving three sorts of memory suited to the process of interpretation: the *continuous past* of the Kleinian that lets itself be recorded in a *memory-file*; the *tendentious past* of the Freudian because it is rewritten at the moment of the Oedipal complex and undergoes successive mutations, thus situations of mourning, which call for various *commemorations* (see *Past* in this glossary). Personally, de M'Uzan subscribes to the latter while nuancing it in an important way, being ever faithful to the economic order, into *cumulative past*. (See "The Person of Myself" [1983a]; "Interpréter: pour qui, pourquoi?" [1983b, 1994b, pp. 69–82]; "Stratégie et tactique à propos des interpretations freudiennes et kleiniennes" [1988, 1994b, pp. 105–114]; "Interpretation and Memory" [1993; this volume].)

Interpretive Darwinism

For de M'Uzan, interpretation behaves like a "living creature".

> Under these conditions, there are grounds for suggesting that the functioning (not the content) of interpretation is subject to the decisive activity of the mechanism that manages the fate of living matter, that is to say, Darwinian selection. The latter is put in the service of the analyst's instruments of thought without, however, undermining the laws of psychic life.

Interpreting is in short remembering. According to de M'Uzan, "the present is the object of a permanent investigation . . . that transforms it tendentiously into the past, which in turn will be commemorated and betrayed". (See "Interpretation and Memory" [1993; this volume].)

Interventions in analysis

Following K.A. Kemper (U.S.A.) and S. Nacht or M. Bouvet in France, de M'Uzan advocates certain specific ways of intervening that stand in contrast to interventions in secondarised language. They must be brief, incomplete and ambiguous in order to stimulate the patient, who is required to complete this singular grammar, by making them his or her own.

This mode of intervention is structured like jokes, dreams or symptoms and is therefore likely to shake up the patient's preconscious, leaving him or her a degree of freedom that is almost creative (see "Interpréter: pour qui, pourquoi?" [de M'Uzan, 1983b; 1994b, pp. 69–82]). Subsequently, having established the necessity for the analyst to think about the unconscious in terms of two orders, that of the psychosexual and that of the vital-identital,* de M'Uzan was to refine further the modalities of interpretation, when the patient finds him- or herself on the axis of self-preservation and its deficiencies, by according a key role to "perceptual activity".

Line of meaning or red line

The organisational factor is mentalisation. Along the line of meaning, on the side of the neuroses, anxiety hysteria separates phobic neurosis and obsessional neurosis, both of which are strongly mentalised. Beneath it we have the actual neuroses (anxiety neurosis, essential depressions, "neurasthenia", somato-functional disorders). On the side of the psychoses, it is depersonalisation* that is located on the line of meaning. Above it, we have the paraphrenias and the delusions of imagination, and beneath it the *actual psychoses* and the somatoses, that is to say, deficiency-based entities whose constitution derives neither from a work of the ego bearing on instinctual drive representations nor from the confrontation with a return of the repressed in the framework of *représentance* (i.e. a general category including different types of representation (psychic representative, ideational representative, affect representative, representative of the drive, etc.). (See "Le développement identitaire: accomplissements et achoppements" [2005b, 2005a, pp. 142–164, 157].)

Masochistic movement

The perverse masochist fears nothing, not even castration, and desires everything, including castration. De M'Uzan nevertheless detects in this type of structure, usually considered as lethal, a possible movement in the direction of a decline in orgastic power thanks to analysis. (See "Un cas de masochisme pervers" [1972, 1977, pp. 125–150].)

Negotiations between two orders of functioning

Having been led to distinguish between two modes of functioning, that of the libidinal, narcissistic and object-related axis, and that of the programme of life with death at the end, the domain of the "*vital-identital*"* in which neither drive activity nor mentalisation have a place, de M'Uzan stresses the need for indispensable "negotiations" between these two orders in every analysis and especially in cases of actual neuroses, actual psychoses and somatoses. (See "Le développement identitaire: accomplissements et achoppements" [2005b]; "Reconsiderations and new developments in psychoanalysis" [2013b, pp. 187–200]; Baruch [2011, p. 47].) In the latter collective work the reader will find after each chapter of an author, the "Response" by de M'Uzan discussing the paper of the author in question.

Operational thinking

Summarised briefly, "operational thinking" (*pensée opératoire*) is a conscious mode of psychic activity, devoid of any links with fantasy activity. This form of psychic activity doubles and illustrates action without really representing it. It develops, in contrast to obsessional thought, within a limited, conformist temporal field without symbolic significance. When we accompany the phenomenon in a subject who invests in a major way in behaviour, we may note that the subject has difficulty in recognising the other as different from him- or herself.

Such a mode of mental functioning is related therefore only to the most concrete aspects of reality. It is marked by a hypercathexis of factual elements and a deficiency in mentalisation. This mode of thinking can be found in patients suffering from somatic, organic or functional illnesses (see Marty & de M'Uzan, 1963; de M'Uzan, Marty, & David, 1963).

In 2005, still concerned by psychosomatics, de M'Uzan wrote:

> Hypercathecting the most concrete aspects of reality "operationally", and by means of tense perception, is one of the conceivable responses to the threat of hallucinatory eruptions of a signifier in consciousness. . . . Operational thinking . . . may be considered . . . as a defence against the consequences of a psychotic defence. We can appreciate here the risk of "psychicizing" in the extreme the pathogenesis of somatic illnesses and, consequently, of attaching to the order of the psychoses somatoses that are often only flanked by operational mental functioning.
>
> (de M'Uzan, 2005b, p. 147ff; 2015, pp. 65–76)

We can notice here a deepening of "operational thinking" in the direction of the domain where the "*vital-identital*"* is operative. Likewise, in an interview between Alain Braconnier and de M'Uzan we can read:

> The eruption that threatens operational thinking is the consequence of the implementation of a powerful and very archaic mechanism of defence, the existence of which I have found in Freud's work, where it is called "*Verwerfung*", and which we find in Lacan's work under the term "foreclosure". Lacanian foreclosure is quite close to the Freudian "*Verwerfung*" and to what I call "rejection", that is to say a particular psychic operation that involves the rejection of a representation. The problem, let me add, is that this "expulsion" is in danger of causing what has been rejected to reappear in a hallucinatory mode, and that to avoid it, the subject clings to and hypercathects everything that is most tangible in reality. It is thus a defence against the consequences (hallucinatory) of a defence (rejection).

(See "Entretien avec E. Braconnier" [2003b]; also, concerning this "original defence against a defence", see "Réponse à Claude Smadja" [2011e, p. 86].)

Paradoxical system

The "paradoxical system" is an original mode of psychic functioning in the analyst. Sometimes the analyst is invaded during the session by strange ideational material, unexpected sentences, abstract formula, colourful images, more or less elaborate reveries, etc. These thoughts, images and words, which produce a sort of momentary sense of alienation in the analyst, correspond to psychic processes occurring in the analysand but which have not yet been detected. The most fundamental characteristic of this phenomenon is that it is in advance in relation *both* to the understanding of the material *and* to the fantasies that the patient is in a position to formulate. (See "Countertransference and Paradoxical System" [1976].)

Paraphrenic twin

The question of the double runs through de M'Uzan's thought from one end to the other, making the vacillation of identity one of the principal modes of his thinking which is dominated by the economic point of view.

An important function of "the uncanny"* and of *"creative upheaval"* (*saisissement créateur*), the invention of the double in key situations of life – birth, mourning, approach of death, work of creation, etc. – finds its legitimacy in one of his last theoretical reflections. De M'Uzan suggests that before separating from the world, the subject must separate from him- or herself. This "self" will thus be capable in extreme situations of stimulating the subject once again in order to enable him or her to link up with the self's intimate being. This double-twin, emanating from an original psychic activity, is the expression of a *work of "personation"* to which one can only gain access subsequently through experiences of depersonalisation* (see de M'Uzan, 1999).

At this point, it is worth recalling that for de M'Uzan, when an interpretation seems to be uttered "by an other", it appears to pertain to the *chimera** or to be *paradoxical* and, for the patient, to emanate practically from *him- or herself*. Under these conditions how could it still meet with immune reactions, with rejections? Uttered by a "double" who, in fact, is simply the "person of him- or herself", the interpretation acquires, in this way, an undeniable *power of conviction*. De M'Uzan's *paraphrenic twin* is thus different both from Bion's (1967) "identical twin" and from Anzieu's (1989) "imaginary twin". Bion's "identical twin" translates the subject's inability to tolerate an object that is not entirely under its control. Anzieu's "imaginary twin" refers to a complementary double.

De M'Uzan's "paraphrenic twin" results from a "complex psychic operation" whereby the "archaic self will be able to emerge from primordial being and forge the beginnings of a distinctive identity" (1999, pp. 104–105). (See "La personne de moi-même" [1983a, 1994b, p. 103]; "Le jumeau paraphrénique ou Aux confins de l'identité" [1999, 2005a, p. 21]; and also the ideas developed by M. Gagnebin in her analysis of S. Beckett and the "Eclipses de l'Ego alter" [Gagnebin, 2011, pp. 179–201].)

Past

It is a weighty question. For de M'Uzan the past is not reconstituted during the sessions, but is *constructed*, and is thus never more than a "fable" reported to an other, a *fiction*.

He was the first, in a conference at the Paris Psychoanalytical Society (see de M'Uzan, 1969) to insist on the fruitful and almost creative character of the falsification of the memories reported to an other, in this instance the psychoanalyst. In a lucid intuition that resulted from the study and practice of literary narrative, de M'Uzan, highlighting the inventive and even creative character of the analytic approach, and thus of interpretation, discovered the field explored by the thinkers of *construction in analysis*, such as Serge Viderman (1970). Referring to Freud's (1937) "Constructions in Analysis", Viderman, for his part, innovated by using the term "construction" no longer in the sense of "deduction" that Freud gave to it, but rather, like de M'Uzan, in the sense of a "creation".

De M'Uzan, once again, adopts a position that is poles apart from a knowledge of the "negative".

Next, this view of the past enables de M'Uzan to distinguish Freudian skill from Kleinian technique. For the "Freudian", the past is merely a *succession of mutations* which, following the paradigm of the Oedipus complex, expresses itself in terms of castration. (See de M'Uzan, 1973, 1977, p. 107.) Now all these mutations constantly imply *experiences of mourning*, and thus commemorations, that is to say tendentious but *creative rewritings* of the past. De M'Uzan writes: "Here, nothing is repeated, everything is done again" (1977, "Avant-propos", p. viii). What about the Kleinian analyst for whom a pre-oedipal situation shapes the Oedipus complex, eradicating the very notion of castration? The dimension of the past seems to change radically. It appears as a memory-file (see de M'Uzan, 1988; 1994b, pp. 110–111). With a fondness for dates, events, clarifications, filiations, Kleinian interpretation clearly rejects any deep reorganisation, which is deemed incompatible. More *tactical*, it is often abundant, responding through a case-by-case approach, whereas Freudian interpretation is moved more by a certain *strategy* that obeys the ambiguities linked to loss and its elaboration. Although it is a tragic process, it seems nonetheless to lead ineluctably to change. The question of the conception of the past therefore guides interpretive modalities.

De M'Uzan proposes, then, three types of past. The "radical" past, in the sense that "it specifies the activities of the subject and circumscribes his truth" (Freudian notion); the "primordial" past which concerns "the re-examination of pregenital experiences and their elaboration depending on the drive-related issues of the moment – one keeps, as it were, the *diary of the past*" (Kleinian notion); and the "cumulative" past, which proposes a "prospective version endowed with an energetic potential" (de M'Uzan's position). Thus he writes: "The present is the object of a permanent investigation, in the quasi-legal sense of the term, transforming it tendentiously into the past, a past that in turn will be commemorated and betrayed" (See "Interpretation and Memory" [1993; this volume].)

Paths of an emerging identity

For de M'Uzan, there are *two* paths towards an emerging identity; one is sexual and the other non-sexual. They both develop concurrently, but at the price of a temporal gap, however minimal, in the emergence of drive activity. "Think simply of the role of education", de M'Uzan writes, "its intervention is necessary so that drive activity (then the unconscious) can emerge and come into being, which implies an anteriority of the '*vital-identital*'" (2011d, p. 48). In other words, two complementary referents which must, not without difficulties, be linked with each other. On the one hand, mentalisation "in the sense that it is understood by the psychosomaticians of the Paris School of Psychosomatics, one of whose most singular and fruitful expressions is the 'paradoxical functioning of the mind'" (2005a, p. 145); and, on the other, self-preservation, in other words "that which, in the development of the human being, proceeds from an essentially genetic programme". Mentalisation, during what de M'Uzan calls a "symbolizing negotiation"* – when this is possible – gives quality to quantity. (See "Le développement identitaire: accomplissements et achoppements" [2005b, 2005a, p. 24, 146, 150]; "Réponse à Catherine Chabert" [2011d, p. 48].)

Perceptual activity

It is through recourse to perceptual activity that de M'Uzan thinks he can help the patient "make the way back" from the dementalised order, riveted solely to the programme of life, to the order of object- and narcissistic-related drive functioning. Here is an example of de M'Uzan's technique (2013b, pp. 192–193; 2015a, p. 118):

> An experienced female colleague told me about an incident that some may find rather banal. The session had finished, but just as she was

> leaving, the patient suddenly turned round and kissed my colleague. Quite overcome, she apologised, saying that she had not been able to stop herself. At first a little troubled, the analyst remained silent and still for a brief moment and then, drawing on her experience, invited her patient to come back into her office. This was perfectly reasonable and, in my view, preferable to resorting to a commonplace statement such as, "We can speak about this in the next session". So they went back into the office, stopped, and stood facing each other. Trying to reassure her patient, the analyst told her that anyone can be overcome by emotion. This basically constituted a sort of exoneration from guilt, the reverse of which is a narcissistic injury, "You're not capable of committing a sin", which aggravates the regression. It would have been more appropriate or more prudent, I think, to leave the affective and erotic dimension momentarily "on the sidelines", as it were, and to enlist the help of perception, which corresponds in the first place to a fundamental phase in the installation of psychic functioning. So I suggested that rather than tranquillising her patient, she could have said, "We both found ourselves standing in front of the door", hoping thereby to participate in the construction of this *"flagstone of identity"* . . . that is indispensable for the development of every psychic apparatus.
>
> (2013b, pp. 192–193)

(See *Aux confins de l'identité* [2005a] and "Reconsiderations and New Developments in Psychoanalysis" [2013b, pp. 192–193]; see also *Flagstone of Identity* in this glossary.)

Permanent disquiet

This state results from a "scandal of identity"* that it is necessary, during the analysis, to trigger and even to aggravate. It is a matter of intervening in the self-preservative *field of identity* (that is, nonsexual and thus not drive-based). Consequently, one must disturb (disorganise), undo, as a reference, what Phyllis Greenacre (1958) described as a sense of uniqueness experienced by an integrated organism able to recognise others without ambiguity.

Ordinarily, psychoanalytic treatment aims to help the patient acquire a certain control of his or her instinctual drive functioning, while allowing for a maximum of satisfaction compatible with reality. According to de M'Uzan, analytic treatment has first and foremost another responsibility. When one has in sight the most authentic aspects of the subject, the liberation of one's most intimate self, it is a matter of making sure he or she has the possibility of arriving at a sense of *permanent disquiet*, that is, of reaching a point where his or her uncertain and random character must appear as a fundamental given of being. "I" must be able to recognise itself as other. (See de M'Uzan, 2009, p. 97.) This "uncertain" and "blurred" character of the subject's being emerged in de M'Uzan's thinking as early as his first texts on the psychological chimera in 1978 and reached its full accomplishment in the thinking of his mature years. The idea of the "dissolution of frontiers" and that of "imbrication" no longer suffice. It is certainly a question for him of an "essential aspect of being". Aware of the discoveries of biology, "where the frontier between the inert and the living is unstable and uncertain", de M'Uzan adopts the "science of indefinite frontiers". And he adds:

> But we will have to accept that beyond its therapeutic project, psychoanalysis gives access to a sense of "permanent disquiet", and that Freud's famous "*Wo es war, soll ich werden*" ("Where id was, there ego shall be") must be replaced by "*Wo ich bin, soll es werden*" ("Where ego is, there id shall be").

(See "Les yeux de Chimène" [1997, 2005a, p. 72]; and, "Reconsiderations and New Developments in Psychoanalysis" [2011b, p. 31; 2013b, pp. 199–200].)

The person of myself

For de M'Uzan,

> the chances of an interpretation being successful are greater when it meets two *obligations*. The first is of an *economic* order. It is important that both in its formulation and its "timing" the interpretation takes full account of the status and the regime of energy in the different psychic systems. The second, I would say, through an extension of meaning, is of an *immune* order.
>
> (1983a, 2013b, p. 52)

Which means that "the interpretation should be homogenous with the Ego, failing which there is a risk that it would not be assimilable" (p. 53). So "for the patient it is as if the interpretation had been proffered by *the person of himself*; that is to say his double – a double that speaks from a transitional area" (1983, 1994b, p. 103), which de M'Uzan calls an everyman's land. (See *Paraphrenic twin* in this glossary.) In his books de M'Uzan gives several clinical sequences of this phenomenon. For example, a woman patient said to him: "No, you don't exist, except through me and in me". (See "The Person of Myself" [1983a].)

Post-analytic illness or the "eyes of Chimene"

For de M'Uzan the "after-analysis (*l'après-analyse*) proceeds from the transference illness, constituting a new illness, the post-analytic illness" or "PAI" (in French "MPA") (2005a, p. 68). And he distinguishes between successful but incomplete analyses and unfinished and incomplete analyses. In the first case, the termination of the analysis constitutes a *phenomenological rupture*: the transference neurosis develops fully from its inauguration to its resolution. The mourning of the analytic situation and of analyst have been accomplished. Each now has their own "identity". In the second case, the termination does not constitute a *phenomenological rupture*. The narcissistic libido continues to displace itself over almost the entire breadth of the "spectrum of identity",* while the unstable aspect of identity tends to continue, as evidenced by the resurgence of phenomena of depersonalisation* or the revival of hypnagogic experiences. De M'Uzan summarises the situation as follows:

> The ego itself, having tasted freedom . . . where primary identification and condensation made it a poet of paradox, a master of metaphor so at ease in formal regression, lets itself be seduced by a strange art of thinking – one that occurs, at certain moments, in the course of the sessions – to the point of maintaining an almost addictive relationship with it, and continuing, always a little, to have the "eyes of Chimene" for it.
>
> (2005a, p. 72)

And he adds:

> We will therefore have to accept the provocative formulation according to which "unfinished and incomplete analyses", those where a phenomenological rupture has not occurred and where, as a result, archaic mechanisms that should no longer exist have been preserved, are those that have the best chances of keeping alive the power of creation.
>
> (ibid., p. 74)

(See "Les yeux de chimène" [de M'Uzan, 1997; 2005a, pp. 64–74]; see also *Spectrum of identity* in this glossary.)

Primordial being

I call *primordial being* a basic state of being of the very earliest stages of life, or rather, a state of being from which both the ego and the

> non-ego in the ego proceed. It is an entity that cannot be perceived distinctly and can only be apprehended globally. It is a "that" of which one would readily speak as if it were a space, with the "where" taking precedence over the "who": a space permeated by enormous quantities of surging energy that only obeys the principle of discharge; a veritable chaos . . . a state of being that is perceptible in the very first phases of the life of a newborn baby.
>
> (de M'Uzan, 1999; 2013b, pp. 104–105)

This fate would be incompatible with the continuation of life if it were not thwarted by object-cathexis, first partial, and before that, and primarily, by a fabulous "discovery", namely, *the creation, the invention of a double, of an authentic twin*. "It is by the creative advent of an *archaic self* and an antagonistic relation with it that the archaic self will be able to emerge from primordial being and forge the beginnings of a distinctive identity" (ibid.). (See *Aux confins de l'identité*, 2005a, pp. 20–21.) (See *Paraphrenic twin* in this glossary.)

Process of affectation

De M'Uzan does not subscribe to the term affect, which is too static for him. By "process of *affectation*", he is describing a *movement* that participates in the discovery that the subject makes of his or her identity, a trajectory during which a phenomenon akin to depersonalisation* plays a central role. It will be noted, once again, that de M'Uzan's thought accords priority to the economic order and, in short, is guided by the concern for an evolution that is always possible. (See "Affect et processus d'affectation" [1970].)

Psychic aphanisis

The term "aphanisis" is borrowed from Ernest Jones, who used it to define the disappearance of sexual desire which, according to him, is more fundamental than the fear of castration (see Jones, 1969, pp. 285–286, 401). De M'Uzan takes up this expression in the context of the analyst's mental functioning in the session and presents one of its dangers, and not the least. The identification of the two protagonists has been taken so far that it no longer pertains to objects, figures, but to modes of functioning which are constantly recreated and give rise to a quasi-immune reaction.

Continuing as if the patient's disunited functioning were the analyst's own, the analyst is led, as a last resort, in order to avoid *psychic aphanisis*, to attack his or her own psychic apparatus or, rather, those of its functions which lead to identification. (See "During the Session" [1989].)

Psychological chimera

The "chimera" (de M'Uzan, 1978a) refers to a sort of new organism arising from the meeting of two unconscious minds, the analysand's and the analyst's; it is a monster that possesses its own modes of functioning. The growth of this fabulous child is affected by various influences from its creators. Some of these are related to the structure of the analysand. But account must also be taken of those that depend on the analyst and which arise from a special disposition for primary identification and a tolerance for experiences of *depersonalisation** (see de M'Uzan, 1978a, pp. 89–98; 1994b, 39, 58; see also Chapter 9 in this volume). For de M'Uzan, the appearance of the *psychological chimera* is a mark of the authenticity of the analysis. Some have sought to see in de M'Uzan's "chimera" links with Ogden's "third person" or "analytic third". But we must not overlook the anteriority of de M'Uzan's notion (1978a) in relation to Ogden's (1999). Furthermore, the background against which his reflections evolved is more of a literary and cultural order, and even poetic (he had already written at this time two volumes of "short stories" in the collection "Metamorphose" (Gallimard): *Les Chiens des rois* (1954) and *Le Rire et la poussière* (1962); and later *Celui-là* (1994a) published by Grasset. Whereas Thomas Ogden belongs to a specific genealogy, Melanie Klein, Bion, and today Ogden's ideas perhaps converge with those of Antonino Ferro in Italy and Béatrice Ithier in France. De M'Uzan "lends" his imaginary world to the patient to the point of risking what he has called "psychic aphanisis"* (de M'Uzan, 1989). It therefore has little to do with the "emotional suffering of the patient that is felt and shared by the analyst" in Ogden's work. For de M'Uzan it is not a matter of transforming the so-called "beta elements into alpha elements", but much more of positioning oneself in specific exchanges with the patient. The analyst and the analysand must each have genuine dispositions that allow them to tolerate measured primary regressions and depersonalisations.* Finally, whereas in de M'Uzan's work the chimera is the stamp of an authentic analysis capable of shifting the accents from the "I" (*Je*) on to what he has called the "spectrum of identity",* Ogden speaks of a "third person", but scarcely develops its implications. De M'Uzan has constantly asserted in his writings that, without the constitution of his "chimera" in the transference/countertransference activity, there can be no true analysis, but only "squiggles" in the manner of Winnicott (psychologist, paediatrician and child psychoanalyst), or "emotional sharing of the undreamed and undreamable", where Ogden even goes as far as to postulate that the analysand must be, at the end of the treatment, almost familiar with the emotional life of his psychoanalyst (!). The whole difference with de M'Uzan stems from Ogden's position inherited first from Klein (for whom projective identification is necessarily massive and thus gives rise to a powerful sway over the patient, then passing through Bion. De M'Uzan, for his part, makes scarcely any appeal to the narrativity and event-based history of the analysand,* which he sees in terms of identifying the particular mental structures of the patient, whereas Ogden regards this as an opportunity for shared reveries with his patient. What interests de M'Uzan, as a psychoanalyst, is the specific character of the patient's mental functioning and of his modes of enunciation (including repressions, avoidances, retroactive undoing, etc.), which he identifies as belonging to the order of a fiction or of a fable reported to another person. (See de M'Uzan, 1989, 1994b, p. 56.) De M'Uzan summarises as follows these different analytic positions concerning the "counter-attitudes" of the psychoanalyst during the session by three terms: egg-laying, covetousness and domination (see *Interpretation* in this glossary). De M'Uzan has little taste for actual stories arising from everyday biography, or recollected stories that arouse in the protagonists an irresistible need to tell each other about their real or mental experiences (Ogden and the predominant role of "projective identification"). Within these same stories of the past related by the patient, what interests de M'Uzan is their rhetoric, their *mise en scène*, which makes a major difference.

To illustrate this, here is a recent clinical example. A woman patient, in a state of great fright, asked herself: "Where am I? Who am I? Everywhere, nowhere". And de M'Uzan comments:

> As soon as the questioning begins – whether as a challenge or out of insouciance – blissful simplicity effaces itself in favour of nowhere and of everywhere. To call into question – and seriously – the hypothetical notion of identity which each of us, without knowing it, believes he or she possesses, great insouciance or great madness is required, but it can happen. Imagine it has happened. Imagine it, close at hand, so to speak, and the drama that then unfolds: "My frontiers are being torn to shreds . . .". The woman who has come to see me in confidence sees a rabbit's head bathed in blood, and in the process of dissolving in a pan. It is a part of herself: "It doesn't belong to me and yet it is me", and she continues, "An unknown zone that is me but does not belong to me. It is as if, continuing to look at this part of myself, this part of myself was going to take precedence over the other part, and then I would be nothing but that". But who is this woman, where is she, this woman, who at other moments is so wise and so reasonable?
>
> (2015a, p. 57; also Chapter 5 in this volume)

At this precise moment in her depersonalisation,* de M'Uzan heard himself say: "Your contours are in my pocket". "On hearing these words, the patient pulled herself together, found the strength to get up off the couch – the session having finished – and to leave. What happened? My intervention, which came naturally from my mouth, corresponded to what I have referred to, since 1978, as the intervention of the 'chimera'" (see de M'Uzan, 2008a).

It is worth noting, however, that the patient, at this moment in the session and the analysis, was profoundly disorganised, having lost her sense of identity usually united within an "I". She saw herself as disseminated along the "spectrum of identity". De M'Uzan's intervention bearing on her destabilising and distressing sense of dissolution ("your contours") had the aim of bringing her back from the self-preservative axis which he called *"vital-identital"** – the programme of life including death at the end, and in which instinctual drive functioning is not involved – to the libidinal, instinctual drive, object-related and narcissistic axis ("you are in 'my' pocket"). It will be understood that this transition from the *vital-identital* to the libidinal sphere implies for the analyst the use of a new grammar. The chimera of de M'Uzan clearly refers to what he has described under the term "paradoxical system",* where the adjective paradoxical does not really suggest the regime that is characteristic of the night dream, and even less the reveries that are allegedly shared between the patient and the analyst, but much more the poetic activity of thought so brilliantly expounded by Antonin Artaud or Andrei Biely.

Rule of "as if/like that"

This is a rule that de M'Uzan follows when he interprets what his patients say, their dreams, memories, slips of the tongue, etc. Affirmatively, he states that things happened *like that*, knowing that a patient's *like that* is only an *as if*, but nothing happens if this *as if* is not taken for an authentic *like that*. (See "Interpretation and Memory" [1993; this volume].)

Same and identical

The repetition of the same and the repetition of the identical do not have the same status for this author.

The first allows for small variations and is creative; the second is deadly. The notion of the past is revisited in the first insofar as it is constantly rewritten, and thus reinvented, something the repetition of the identical fails to investigate. (See de M'Uzan, 1969.) This chapter ("The Same and the Identical") has become a reference in the history of psychoanalysis. The work of de M'Uzan is not only known in France but also in England, America, Germany and Spain, where his books and in particular this article have often been translated. (See 2013b, 2014a, 2014b, 2004b, pp. 23–25.)

Scandal of identity

This term refers to an economic scandal provoked in the higher psychic systems, making it possible to put psychic energy back into circulation where it has been immobilised by the regime of binding. Without this scandal of identity, it would not be possible for any interpretation to be cathected except in the form of a factor aggravating resistance. (See "Du derangement au changement" [1991, 1994b, pp. 115–128].)

Silence of the psychoanalyst or the mouth of the unconscious

The analyst's silence plays a role in establishing a climate of strangeness, which is an indication that issues of identity are involved. Here we are touching on the analyst's power, which is considerable and even at the limits of what is acceptable. De M'Uzan calls this silence, which is equally the lever of the patient's projections and has nothing to do with mutism, "the mouth of the unconscious". (See "The Mouth of the Unconscious" [1978a; this volume]; and "Introduction to the Theory of the Preliminary Interview" [2010; this volume].)

Spectrum of identity

The spectrum of identity indicates the variable positions adopted by the analyst and the analysand in the area of transition which, created in the course of the session, both separates and links them. It is in this zone where the frontiers between the ego and the non-ego are more than uncertain, and whose constitution attests, in both protagonists, to a disposition for primary identification, that the famous *chimera** is formed. It seems to de M'Uzan that the definition of the sense of identity advanced by Phyllis Greenacre (1958), who defends the sense of uniqueness experienced by an integrated organism that is able to recognise others without ambiguity needs to be termed less rigidly. (See de M'Uzan, 1983a; 1994b, p. 98; 2013b, p. 61.) In fact, for him,

> if "I" is not in the ego, it not entirely in the other either, but distributed along the fringes of a spectrum, let us say of a spectrum of identity defined by all the various positions that the narcissistic libido can adopt; or, more precisely, by the places and quantities cathected by the narcissistic libido, extending from an inner pole to an outer pole that coincides with the image of the other.

(See "If I Were Dead" [1974a, 1978b].)

Strategy and tactics

These are the two modes of interpretation according to de M'Uzan. Tactics is the favoured mode of the Kleinians who follow what their patients say step by step and respond in kind. He writes: "The Kleinian analyst, who follows the transference movements as closely as possible, has a great deal of operational flexibility. He or she is, as it were 'in contact'". Both the opposition good/bad (the binary mode therefore) and the extensive recourse to the role of projection confronting two subjects caught in their reality, attest to "a very affirmative, selective and concentrated style . . . that offers truly tactical support" (1988, 1994b, p. 106). We are reminded of the "habitual generosity of the Kleinian discourse". The step-by-step approach that, according to de M'Uzan, characterises Kleinian intervention/interpretation, stands in contrast to the Freudian strategy which develops by according an eminent role to castration and thus to the Oedipus complex which cancels out the Kleinian necessity for a pre-oedipal stage. For de M'Uzan everything is played out with the discovery of the Oedipus complex and, consequently, the past is rewritten. Such a mode of interpretation, presupposes, as in chess, a plan in the meanderings of interpretation.

> Kleinian fear and destructiveness is matched by ideas of laws and prohibitions; the tension between good and bad and direct instinctual drive aims are thwarted by the tendentious account of a necessarily mediated desire, as it is expressed in a complex drama comprising at least three characters.
>
> (1994b, p. 107)

The ternary mode, the relationship with time, ideas of waiting and of position, and temporisation with silence (which is not mutism) have the effect that when the time comes "interpretation is no longer limited to formulating *contents*, but relationships" (ibid.).

The step-by-step and affirmative work of the Kleinian is to be distinguished from the "interpretive *periods*" of the Freudian analyst. De M'Uzan adheres to the latter. (See "Stratégie et tactique à propos des interprétations freudiennes et kleiniennes" [1988, 1994b, pp. 105–114]; see also *Interpretation* in this glossary.)

Therapeutic indications

For de M'Uzan, borderline cases are the best therapeutic indications. In 1977, he wrote: "It is in states without limits, where the 'oedipal' verb ceases to be conjugated, that the human being can find the means to change himself into an oeuvre to be completed" (de M'Uzan, 1977, p. x). His concern for the economic dimension and his "artistic" vision of analysis can be recognised here. (Concerning the "artistic" view of analysis in de M'Uzan's work, see Gagnebin, 1996.)

Trajectory of bisexuality

In de M'Uzan's work, bisexuality corresponds "to the integration of the male and female elements" following the alternate rhythm of progressive and retrogressive movements. Thus psychic bisexuality has to be *earned*; it is the end of an evolution whose course is irregular and difficult, always in danger of coming to a standstill. It is a demand for work imposed on the psychic apparatus and, as such, it can be likened to a creative process. It must not be confused with androgyny (a "biological monster" endowed with both sexes) nor with ambisexuality where the subject lives out sexuality with the representatives of both sexes. Once again, bisexuality is always psychic. (See "Trajectoire de la bisexualité" [1975, 1977, pp. 113–122].)

Transference neurosis

This key moment in analysis is considered as a *novel* and differs from the simple transferences that are met with in life. As a novel, analysis has a trajectory and, consequently, an end. De M'Uzan develops his conception of a past that is always tendentious, rewritten for an other (the analyst), and thus partly fictive and definitely *fictional*. (See "Transferts et névrose de transfert" [1966, 1977, pp. 67–74].)

Transitional subject

D.W. Winnicott used the term "transitional object" to refer to the object that the child chooses (teddy, handkerchief, blankets, and today he would no doubt have added the famous "stuffed toys"); an object that represents both the child and the mother, while at the same time being also the bear, handkerchief or blanket. For Winnicott, the child will one day abandon, quite naturally, this transitional object, having succeeded in differentiating between the different beings. If the child is unable to leave it, he or she will transform the transitional object into a "fetish object" and the field of perversions will then be opened up. (See Winnicott [1971] and the concept of "potential space".)

Based on this model, André Green (1992) put forward the term "transnarcissistic object" for the work of art that speaks to individuals at a level that goes beyond their purely personal preoccupations. He thus considers that the foundations for creative work lie beyond a simple narcissistic projection of the artist.

The "transitional subject" is something quite different for de M'Uzan. It refers to the very first stages of individuation.

> Before progressing in the acquisition of its own identity, drawing on an antagonism with the non-self by way of support, the archaic self must first differentiate itself from itself. . . . This archaic self, the essence of the future subject, first has the task of emerging from an indistinct syncretic entity that I call *primordial being*, a basic state of being of the very earliest stages of life, or rather, a state of being from which both the ego and the non-ego in the ego proceed. . . . It is a "that" of which one would readily speak as if it were a space, with the *where* taking precedence over the *who*; a space permeated by enormous quantities of surging energies that only obey the principle of discharge; a veritable chaos, which can be found, moreover, albeit in a different way, in the field of the drives when no overall organisation has been able to impose itself. It is a state of being that is perceivable in the very first phases of the life of a newborn baby. Such a fate would be incompatible with the continuation of life or, more precisely, with the accomplishment of the genetic programme in the service of which the drives are employed, if it were not thwarted, as we know, by the object-cathexis at first partial, and before that by a fabulous "discovery": *the creation, the invention of a double, of an authentic twin*. . . . A complex psychical operation is involved because it is by virtue of the creative advent of a twin and an antagonistic relationship with it that the *archaic self* will be able to emerge from primordial being and forge the beginnings of a distinctive identity. This double/twin, emanating from primordial psychic activity, is the expression of a work of *"personation"* to which one can only gain access subsequently during experiences of depersonalisation.
>
> (de M'Uzan, 1999; 2005a, pp. 20–21; 2013b, pp. 104–105)

While Winnicott's transitional phenomenon has an undeniable external materiality, preparing for the full cathexis of the object, de M'Uzan's *transitional subject* is "a psychic being whose place and nature can be inferred from the traces that remain of it throughout the individual's history" (2013b, pp. 105–106). This elementary self, edifying itself with the help of the intervention of a double has no need to differentiate itself from a *non-ego* on the path to objectalisation. It emanates purely from itself and thus differs from the world of objects, narcissistic objects included. It is charged with an energy that comes not from the British "no man's land" but from an "every man's land". In the place of the British nothing, de M'Uzan proposes an everything. That is why, for this analyst, the establishment of the first strata of the status of identity must take place under the authority of the forces of self-preservation insofar as they are opposed to the sexual drives. (See de M'Uzan, *Aux confins de l'identité*, 2005a, pp. 17–24; *Michel de M'Uzan ou le saisissement créateur*, Gagnebin & Milly, 2012, p. 183; see also *vital-identital* in this glossary.)

The Uncanny

It was in 1919, in *Imago*, that Freud (1919h) first used this complex notion to highlight a psychic state, a sensation or a feeling caused by the resurgence of a repressed object or situation that was cathected and even familiar in childhood. Their reappearance procures a new perception that gives them an aspect of strangeness, of being almost unfamiliar, capable of giving rise to various feelings of terror. In general, the sense of uncanniness is linked to the notions of "déjà *vu*" or "déjà *entendu*". It is operative in infantile reminiscences that had once been repressed owing to the child's immaturity. Its territories of choice are also the artistic domain and the literary field. Freud, then, traces the experience of the uncanny back to the return of the repressed and castration anxiety. In "A Disturbance of Memory on the Acropolis", Freud (1936) admits that he might have had a momentary feeling that what he saw was not real. He points out that "such a feeling is known as a 'feeling of derealisation' (*Entfremdungsgefühl*)." He states elsewhere that it is marked by the fact that

> the subject identifies himself with someone else, so that he is in doubt as to which his self is, or substitutes the extraneous self for his own. In other words, there a doubling, a dividing, and interchanging of the self.
>
> (Freud, 1919h, p. 234)

When de M'Uzan uses this notion, he gives priority to the term *strangeness* (*étrangété*). For him it is an impression that becomes stronger each time that natural distinctions tend to disappear: distinctions between the inside and the outside, the ego and the non-ego, the subject and the object, the familiar and the unfamiliar. Consequently, for this psychoanalyst, as the uncanny does not tolerate being confined within a too restricted notional framework, it will become the support for a *relationship* in which *what is disturbing* and *what is fascinating* are opposed. In other words, the phenomenon characterises a natural status of the frontiers of being that have become mobile and, as a result, favour "psychization", that is to say an inscription in the psychosexual register, with objectalisation in view. The uncanny is clearly located at the crossroads of the two orders that de

M'Uzan has defined, that of the object- and narcissistic-related libidinal *drive axis* and that of the programme characteristic of the *vital-identital,** one of the moments of which is self-preservation. The uncanny constitutes a key activity of the "negotiation"* between these two orders. (See "The Uncanny or 'I Am Not Who You Think I Am'" [2009]. See also *Vital-identital* in this glossary.)

Vacillation of identity

The theme of identity runs through de M'Uzan's theoretical thinking from one end to the other. He considers that identity, a major theme in his work, must be led, through analysis, to a state of vacillation so that something can change in the subject. The constitution of a "double", or of a "paraphrenic twin", which is so important for this author, is a provisional solution to the vacillation of identity advocated by de M'Uzan. The theme of identity is therefore for him not part of some kind of normative aim, but acquires the significance of putting psychic energy back into circulation that is liable to bring about the reorganisations necessary for change. Identity is thus strongly bound up with the "economic" question as explored by Freud in his metapsychology, and which de M'Uzan logically espouses in his own work. He even goes as far as to propose the notion of "transitional subject" echoing D.W. Winnicott's "transitional object". (See among other texts: "Countertransference and Paradoxical System" [1976b]; "The Mouth of the Unconscious" [1978a; this volume]; "During the Session" [1989]; "The Paraphrenic Twin or at the Frontiers of Identity" [1999]; "Séparation et identité" [2001a], and "Le développement identitaire: accomplissements et achoppements" [2005b]. See also *Transitional subject* in this glossary.)

Vital-identital

This is a fundamental concept in de M'Uzan's theory; indeed, it is one of his revolutionary contributions. It corresponds to an order of identity that stands in contrast to sexual drive functioning (object- and narcissistic-related). Concerning this order one could readily speak of a real *programme* of life, and thus of death at the end. The classical notion of *self-preservation* is part of it. Along this axis of identity, mentalisation is deficient. The "neurotic" dimension is not involved. Consequently, we find ourselves at the heart of the actual neuroses and equally of the actual psychoses. The term drive does not have its place in this order. After making a clear distinction between the order of the *"vital-identital"* and that of psychosexuality, de M'Uzan explains how the analyst must know how to resort to *negotiations** between these two axes in such a way as to help the patient find his or her way back to the psychosexual order and avoid somatoses or actual neuroses, or even actual psychoses. De M'Uzan created the neologism *"vital-identital"*, first as an echo to the notion of the *sexual* elaborated by Jean Laplanche, whose views on this subject he shares, and secondly to distinguish it from the concept of identity which pertains to the philosophical domain. (See *Aux confins de l'identité* [2005a] and "Reconsiderations and New developments in Psychoanalysis" [2011, p. 24ff.; 2013b, p. 192ff.]; see also Gagnebin & Milly [2012, p. 182].)

Work of dying

De M'Uzan insists on the individual's specific capacities of life and creation when faced with death. Using simultaneously the specific resources of depersonalisation, of the paradoxical, of dissociation, and even of the emergence of a "paraphrenic twin",* the individual, *thanks to analytic work*, tries, one last time, to put him- or herself totally in the world. (See "The Work of Dying" [1977b] and "Last Words" [1981; this volume].)

***

The fifty notions in this glossary highlight not only de M'Uzan's analytic creativity and generosity, but also his thinking that is radically oriented towards the self-creation of the individual, a process that is always possible and renewable right up until the moment of dying.

However, the metapsychological revolution introduced by de M'Uzan revolves around the invention of two analytic axes: the psychosexual axis on the one hand and the programme of life with death at the end on the other; that is to say, where the *"vital-identital"** plays a part both in the indispensable constitution of the *"flagstone of identity"** and in its deficiencies that undermine the sense of identity. These extremely painful deficiencies are an indication of sufferings caused by intolerable experiences of incapacity in the individual.

This invention of two psychic orders that are separated by greater or lesser capacities for mentalisation, is without doubt the most important metapsychological revolution introduced by de M'Uzan.

Awareness of castration or of the non-omnipotence of humankind only exists on the psychosexual axis – the axis that generally is given priority in psychoanalysis – as does access to psychic mutations and thus to creativity. The axis of the *"vital-identital"*, ensuring the programme of life with death at the end is nonetheless absolutely necessary for the formation of the "flagstone of identity". However, when "actual energy" is perverted, this same *"vital-identital"* leads directly to the somatoses, to the "actual neuroses", and to the "actual psychoses". The distinction between these two orders is a discovery arising from clinical experience and compensates for a lack in the systemic Unconscious, which constitutes a considerable advance at the metapsychological level. The most essential idea of de M'Uzan concerns a task that is incumbent upon the analyst. The analyst must be able to *negotiate* between the two axes with the patient in order to help the patient to get back above the "line of meaning",* which means relearning to mentalise conflicts until she or he is able to get beyond them – a new sort of creation.

De M'Uzan, then, is fascinated by questions of identity and this has been the case ever since his first experiences in psychosomatic medicine right up until their current elaboration in a revisited metapsychology.

The dominant idea is that the individual is fundamentally capable of psychic mutations thanks to analytic work which (1) knows how to listen to the two axes: namely, the psychosexual and the *"vital-identital"*,* whose *negotiations** he or she explores. This involves new modes of intervention. As a result, interpretation can be assimilated by the patient who experiences it as coming from *him- or herself*; and (2) authorises both analyst and patient alike to develop, without fear, primary regressions and depersonalisations,* where the patient feels so closely bound up with the analyst that the patient no longer knows who is who.

Furthermore, de M'Uzan never gives up, even when it comes to the "work of dying",* offering his analysands the possibility of working psychically – insofar as they can – and to continue their self-engenderment until the end.

We can see how for more than sixty years the economic dimension has remained for this thinker of psychoanalysis the essential factor of analytic work, favouring psychic disruptions and mutations, which he calls a state of "permanent disquiet".* He is a discrete thinker who places his trust in *silence* – and not the mutism of the interpreter – which he calls "the mouth of the unconscious"; he thereby places value on the work that is taken up over and over again, and that is inspired by the attraction of the analytic exercise that he calls "the eyes of Chimene".*

In short, he is a thinker of the economic dimension in the analytic sense of the term, a thinker who has faith in psychic changes and is therefore persuaded that they can bring about an undeniable deliverance for the patient. He is a thinker who listens to the psychosexual order of functioning, but is also attentive to the continuous bass of the *"vital-identital"*. The energy of the latter is often degraded and requires of the analyst a genuine tolerance for primary regression and for depersonalisation* experienced almost to the point of "psychic aphanisis".* Finally, he is a psychoanalytic thinker whose theoretical developments are always based on his own clinical experiences.

De M'Uzan has not sought to compete with other doctrines, preferring to devote himself entirely to listening to his patients in a *lively* manner, which is without doubt the best school and the finest adventure!

Note

1 Contrary to conventions, the author's name is written: de M'Uzan.

References

Allègre, C. (1992). *Introduction à une histoire naturelle*. Paris: Fayard.

Anzieu, D. (1989). Beckett et Bion. *Revue française de psychanalyse*, 53(5): pp. 1405–1415.

Artaud, A. (1947). Artaud le mômo, Vol. XII. Paris: Bordas. Reprinted in *Oeuvres completes*. Paris: Gallimard, 1974. [Artaud the Mômo. In B. Bador (trans.), *Watchfiends and rackscreams, works from the final period*, New York, NY: Exact Exchange Press, 1995.]

Ascher, J., & Jouet, J. P. (2004). *La Greffe, entre biologie et psychanalyse*. Preface by M. de M'Uzan. Paris: Presses Universitaires de France.

Barthes, R. (1953). *Writing degree zero* (trans. Annette Lavers, & Colin Smith). Preface by Susan Sontag. New York, NY: Beacon Press, 1970.

Barthes, R. (1964). L'écrivain et l'écrivant. In *Essais Critiques, Œuvres Complètes*, 1: pp. 1277–1282.

Baruch, C. (ed.) (2011). *Nouveaux développements en psychanalyse. Autour de la pensée de Michel de M'Uzan*. Sèvres: EDK.

Biely, A. (1915). *Kotik Letaev* (trans. G. J. Janecek). Evanston, IL: Northwestern University Press, 1999.

Bion, W. R. (1967). *Second thoughts*. London: Heinemann.

Bouvet, M. (1960). Dépersonnalisation et relations d'objet. In *Oeuvres psychanalytiques 1, La relation d'objet: Névrose obsessionnelle, dépersonnalisation*. Paris: Presses Universitaires de France, pp. 295–435.

Chantoiseau, J. B. (ed.) (2014). *L'En-deça des images: Autour de l'oeuvre de Murielle Gagnebin*. Seyssel: Champ Vallon.

Charon, J. E. (1977). *L'esprit, cet inconnu*. Paris: Albin Michel.

David, C. (1996). Le deuil de soi-même. *Revue française de psychanalyse*, 60(1): pp. 15–32.

M'Uzan, M. de (1954). *Les chien des rois*. Paris: Gallimard.

M'Uzan, M. de (1962). *Le rire et la poussière*. Paris: Gallimard.

M'Uzan, M. de (1965). Aperçus sur le processus de la création littéraire. *Revue française de psychanalyse*, 29(1): pp. 43–64; also in de M'Uzan, 1977: pp. 3–27.

M'Uzan, M. de (1966). Transferts et névrose de transfert. *Revue française de psychanalyse*, 32(2): pp. 235–245; also in de M'Uzan, 1977: pp. 67–74.

M'Uzan, M. de (1967). Acting out 'direct' et acting out 'indirect', paper read at the 28th Congress for French-speaking Psychoanalysts in 1967 on the Report by Julien Rouart: "Agir et processus analytique", *Revue française de psychanalyse*, 32(5–6): pp. 995–1000; also in de M'Uzan, 1977a: pp. 75–82.

M'Uzan, M. de (1968). Freud et la mort. *L'Arc*, 34: pp. 55–66; also in de M'Uzan, 1977: pp. 49–63.

M'Uzan, M. de (1969). Le même et l'identique. *Revue française de psychanalyse*, 3: pp. 441–451; also in de M'Uzan, 1977: pp. 83–97. First published in English in the *Psychoanalytic Quarterly*, 76: pp. 1205–1220 and republished in de M'Uzan, 2013b: pp. 3–16.

M'Uzan, M. de (1970). Affect et processus d'affectation, *Revue française de psychanalyse*, 34(5–6): pp. 1197–1202; also in de M'Uzan, 1977: pp. 98–105.

M'Uzan, M. de (1972). Un cas de masochisme pervers: Esquisse d'une théorie. In J. McDougall (ed.), *La sexualité perverse*. Paris: Payot; also in de M'Uzan, 1977: pp. 125–150.

M'Uzan, M. de (1973). Notes sur l'évolution et la nature de l'Idéal du Moi. *Revue française de psychanalyse*, 37(5–6): pp. 1014–1018; also in de M'Uzan, 1977: pp. 106–112.

M'Uzan, M. de (1974a). "S.j.e.m." Le dehors et le dedans. *Nouvelle revue de psychanalyse*, 9: pp. 23–32. [(1978). If I were dead. *International Review of Psychoanalysis*, 5: pp. 485–490.]

M'Uzan, M. de (1974b). Psychodynamic mechanisms in psychosomatic symptom-formation. *Psychotherapy and Psychosomatics*, 23(1–6): pp. 103–110. (Acts of the 2nd Congress of Psychosomatic Medicine, Amsterdam, 1973).

M'Uzan, M. de (1974c). Analytical process and the notion of the past. *International Review of Psychoanalysis*, 74(1): pp. 461–466.

M'Uzan, M. de (1975). Trajectoire de la bisexualité. *Revue française de psychanalyse*, 39(5–6): pp. 885–892; also in de M'Uzan, 1977: pp. 113–122.

M'Uzan, M. de (1976a). Le travail du trépas. In M. de M'Uzan (ed.), 1977, pp. 182–199. English translation in de M'Uzan, 2013b: pp. 33–46.

M'Uzan, M. de (1976b). Contre-transfert et système paradoxal. *Revue française de psychanalyse*, 40(3): pp. 575–590; also in de M'Uzan, 1977: pp. 164–181. English translation in de M'Uzan, 2013b: pp. 17–32.

M'Uzan, M. de (1977). *De l'art à la mort*. Paris: Gallimard.

M'Uzan, M. de (1978a). La bouche de l'inconscient. *Nouvelle revue de psychanalyse*, 17: pp. 89–98; also in de M'Uzan, 1994b: pp. 33–44. English translation, Chapter 9 in this volume.

M'Uzan, M. de (1978b). If I were dead. *International Review of Psychoanalysis*, 5: pp. 485–490.

M'Uzan, M. de (1981). Dernières paroles. *Nouvelle revue de psychanalyse*, 23(1): pp. 117–130; also in de M'Uzan, 1994: pp. 13–32. English translation, Chapter 8 in this volume.

M'Uzan, M. de (1983a). La personne de moi-même. *Nouvelle revue de psychanalyse*, 28, pp. 193–208; also in de M'Uzan, 1994b: pp. 83–104. English translation in de M'Uzan, 2013b: pp. 49–66.

M'Uzan, M. de (1983b). Interpréter: Pour qui, pourquoi? *Revue française de psychanalyse*, 47(3): pp. 793–804; also in de M'Uzan, 1994b: pp. 69–82.

M'Uzan, M. de (1984). Les esclaves de la quantité. *Nouvelle revue de psychanalyse*, 30: pp. 129–138; also in de M'Uzan 1994b: pp. 155–168. English translation in de M'Uzan, 2013b: pp. 67–78.

M'Uzan, M. de (1988). Stratégie et tactique à propos des interpretations freudiennes et kleiniennes. *Revue française de psychanalyse*, 52(3): pp. 657–664; also in de M'Uzan, 1994b: pp. 105–114.

M'Uzan, M. de (1989). Pendant la séance. *Nouvelle revue de psychanalyse*, 40: pp. 147–163; also in de M'Uzan, 1994b: pp. 45–68. English translation in de M'Uzan, 2013b: pp. 79–97.

M'Uzan, M. de (1991). Du derangement au changement. *Revue française de psychanalyse*, 55(2): pp. 325–337; also in de M'Uzan, 1994: pp. 115–128.

M'Uzan, M. de (1993). Interprétation et mémoire. *Revue française de psychanalyse*, 57(1): pp. 7–20; also in de M'Uzan, 1994b: pp. 176–183. English translation, Chapter 10 in this volume.

M'Uzan, M. de (1994a). *Celui-là*. Paris: Grasset.

M'Uzan, M. de (1994b). *La Bouche de l'inconscient*. Paris: Gallimard.

M'Uzan, M. de (1996). La mort n'avoue jamais. *Revue française de psychanalyse*, 60(1): pp. 33–47; also in 2005: pp. 41–63. English translation in de M'Uzan, 2013b: pp. 119–235.

M'Uzan, M. de (1997). Les yeux de Chimène. *Revue française de psychanalyse*, 61(4): pp. 1113–1120; also in de M'Uzan, 2005a: pp. 64–74.

M'Uzan, M. de (1999). Le jumeau paraphrénique ou Aux confins de l'identité. *Revue Française de Psychanalyse*, 63(4): pp. 1135–1151; also in de M'Uzan, 2005a: pp. 15–40. English translation in de M'Uzan, 2013b: pp. 101–118.

M'Uzan, M. de (2001a). Separation et identité. *Revue française de psychanalyse*, 65:pp. 355–360; also in de M'Uzan, 2005: pp. 124–131.

M'Uzan, M. de (2001b). À l'Horizon: Le facteur actuel. *Revue française de psychanalyse* (Courants de la psychanalyse contemporaine, special edition): pp. 335–441; also in 2005a: pp. 113–123.

M'Uzan, M. de (2003a). De l'informe avant toute chose. *Penser/Rêver*, 4, *L'Informe*: pp. 27–36; also in de M'Uzan, 2005a: pp. 100–109.

M'Uzan, M. de (2003b). "Entretien" avec A. Braconnier. *Carnet Psy*, 84(7): pp. 28–33.

M'Uzan, M. de (2004a). Addiction et problématique identitaire: Le 'tonus de base'. *Revue française de psychanalyse*, 65(2): pp. 591–597; also in de M'Uzan, 2005a: pp. 132–141.

M'Uzan, M. de (2004b). Lo mismo y lo identico. In J. F. Artaloytia (trans.), *Revista de Psicoanálisis*: pp. 23–25.

M'Uzan, M. de (2005a). *Aux confins de l'identité*. Paris: Gallimard.

M'Uzan, M. de (2005b). Le développement identitaire: Accomplissements et achoppements. in *Aux confins de l'identité*. Paris: Gallimard, pp. 142–164.

M'Uzan, M. de (2006). Invite à frequenter les ombres. *European Federation of Psychoanalysis Bulletin*, 60: pp. 15–29. English translation de M'Uzan, 2013b: pp. 147–165.

M'Uzan, M. de (2008a). La relation d'objet: Entre qui, entre quoi? Pour qui, pour quoi? In *Annuel de L'Association psychanalytique de France. L'objet, la réalité*. Paris: Presses Universitaires de France; also in 2015: pp. 83–100. English translation in de M'Uzan, 2013b: pp. 169–185.

M'Uzan, M. de (2008b). Une perspective nouvelle en psychanalyse. *Bulletin du Groupe Méditerranéen de la Société Psychanalytique de Paris*, 17: pp. 9–17; also in 2015a: pp. 65–76. English translation, Chapter 6 in this volume.

M'Uzan, M. de (2008c). L'enfer de la créativité. In : McDougall, 2008: pp. 35–46; also in 2015a, pp. 33–42. English translation, this volume Chapter 2.

M'Uzan, M. de (2009). L'inquiétante étrangété ou "Je ne suis pas celle que vous croyez". in *Inquiétante étrangété* ("Monographies et débats de psychanalyse"): pp. 89–98; also in de 2015: pp. 101–111. English translation in de M'Uzan, 2013: pp. 137–146.

M'Uzan, M. de (2010). *Introduction à la théorie de l'entretien préliminaire*. In de M'Uzan (ed.), 2015a: pp. 77–82. English translation, Chapter 7 in this volume.

M'Uzan, M. de (2011a). La corrida . . . et en deçà. *Revue française de psychanalyse*, 75(1): pp. 13–15; also in 2015a: pp. 50–53. English translation, Chapter 4 in this volume.

M'Uzan, M. de (2011b). Reconsidérations et nouveaux développements en psychanalyse. In Baruch, 2011: pp. 17–31; also in 2015a: pp. 112–127. English translation in de M'Uzan, 2013b: pp. 187–200.

M'Uzan, M. de (2011c). Réponse à Clarisse Baruch. In Baruch, 2011: pp. 137–143.

M'Uzan, M. de (2011d). Réponse à Catherine Chabert. In Baruch, 2011: pp. 45–50.

M'Uzan, M. de (2011e). Réponse à Claude Smadja. In Baruch, 2011: pp. 83–88.

M'Uzan, M. de (2011f). Réponse à Sylvie Faure-Pragier. In Baruch, 2011: pp. 71–73.

M'Uzan, M. de (2011g). Problématique identitaire et psychose. *Psychanalyse et Psychose*, 11: pp. 17–23 (Centre de psychanalyse et de psychothérapie J. E. Kestemberg).

M'Uzan, M. de (2012). Le saisissement créateur. In M. Gagnebin & J. Milly (ed.), *Michel de M'Uzan ou le saisissement créateur*. Seyssel: Champ Vallon; also in 2015a: pp. 43–49. English translation, this volume Chapter 3.

M'Uzan, M. de (2013a). Sur les frontières. *Revue française de psychosomatique*, 43: pp. 23–31; also in 2015a: pp. 57–64. English translation, Chapter 5 in this volume.

M'Uzan, M. de (2013b). *Death and identity: Being and the psycho-sexual drama* (trans. Andrew Weller). London: Karnac.

M'Uzan, M. de (2014a). *Identität und Tod* (trans. H. D. Gondek). Giessen: Psychosozial-Verlag.

M'Uzan, M. de (2014b). *Depersonnalisation und Kreativität* (trans. H. D. Gondek). Giessen: Psychosozial-Verlag.

M'Uzan, M. de (2015). *L'inquiétude permanente*. Paris: Gallimard.

M'Uzan, M. de, Marty, P., & David, C. (1963). *L'investigation psychosomatique: Sept observations cliniques* (2nd edition in 1994 (republished in 2015) including "Préliminaires critiques à la recherché psychosomatique" in collaboration with Ch. David).

M'Uzan, M. de, & Pontalis, J. B. (1977). Redirect, psychanalyser, écrire. *Nouvelle revue de psychanalyse*, 16: pp. 5–26.

Donnet, J., & de M'Uzan, M. (1998). La rencontre analytique (Interview by Christine Bouchard and Jean-Michel Porte). *Revue française de psychanalyse*, 62(1): pp. 189–208.

Edelman, G. (1978). *The mindful brain, with V. Mountcastle*. Cambridge, MA: MIT Press.

Edelman, G. (1992). *Bright air, brilliant fire: On the matter of mind*. New York, NY: Basic Books.

Freud, E. L. (ed.) (1960). *Letters of Sigmund Freud, 1873–1939*. London: Hogarth; New York, NY: Basic Books.

Freud, S. (1912). *Recommendations to physicians practising psychoanalysis*. *S.E.* 12. London: Hogarth, pp. 11–120.

Freud, S. (1913). *On beginning the treatment*. *S.E.* 12. London: Hogarth, pp. 123–144.

Freud, S. (1914). *On narcissism: An introduction*. *S.E.* 14. London: Hogarth, pp. 69–102.

Freud, S. (1915a). *Instincts and their vicissitudes. S.E.* 14. London: Hogarth, pp. 109–140.

Freud, S. (1915b). *The unconscious. S.E.* 14. London: Hogarth, pp. 166–215.

Freud, S. (1917). *A difficulty in the path of psychoanalysis. S.E.* 17. London: Hogarth, pp. 137–144.

Freud, S. (1919a [1918]). *Lines of advance in psycho-analytic therapy. S.E.* 17. London: Hogarth, pp. 159–168.

Freud, S. (1919b). *The "Uncanny". S.E.* 17. London: Hogarth, pp. 217–252.

Freud, S. (1920). *Beyond the pleasure principle. S.E.* 18. London: Hogarth, pp. 1–64.

Freud, S. (1923). *The ego and the id. S.E.* 19. London: Hogarth, pp. 3–66.

Freud, S. (1926). *Inhibitions, symptoms and anxiety. S.E.* 20. London: Hogarth, pp. 75–174.

Freud, S. (1936). *A disturbance of memory on the Acropolis. S.E.*, 22. London: Hogarth, pp. 239–250.

Freud, S. (1937a). *Analysis terminable and interminable. S.E.* 23. London: Hogarth, pp. 209–253.

Freud, S. (1937b). *Constructions in analysis. S.E.* 23. London: Hogarth, pp. 255–269.

Freud, S. (1939). *Moses and monotheism. S.E.* 23. London: Hogarth, pp. 1–137.

Freud, S. (1940). *An outline of psychoanalysis. S.E.* 23. London: Hogarth, pp. 139–207.

Freud, S. (1950 [1895]). *Project for a scientific psychology. S.E.* 1. London: Hogarth, pp. 281–397.

Freud, S. (1991). *Gesammelte Werke.* Frankfurt am Main: Fischer.

Freud, S., & Breuer, J. (1895). *Studies on hysteria. S.E.* 2. London: Hogarth.

Gagnebin, M. (1996). *Michel de M'Uzan.* Paris: Presses Universitaires de France.

Gagnebin, M. (2004). *Authenticité du faux, lectures psychanalytiques.* Paris: Presses Universitaires de France.

Gagnebin, M. (2011). *En deça de la sublimation: L'Ego alter.* Paris: Presses Universitaires de France.

Gagnebin, M., & Milly, J. (2012). *Michel de M'Uzan ou le saisissement créateur.* Seyssel: Champ Vallon.

Green, A. (1980). The dead mother. In Andrew Weller (trans), *Life narcissism, death narcissism.* London: Free Association Books, pp. 170–200.

Green, A. (1983). *Life narcissism, death narcissism* (trans. Andrew Weller). London: Free Association Books, 2001.

Green, A. (1990a). Remémoration: effet de mémoire ou temporalité à l'oeuvre. *Revue française de psychanalyse*, 4: pp. 947–972.

Green, A. (1990b). Temps et mémoire. *Nouvelle revue de psychanalyse*, 41: pp. 179–205.

Green, A. (1992). *La déliaison: psychanalyse, anthropologie et literature.* Paris: Hachette.

Green, A., & Donnet, J. L. (1973). *L'Enfant de Ca: psychanalyse d'un entretien: La psychose blanche.* Paris: Minuit.

Greenacre, P. (1958). *Emotional growth*, Vols 1 & 2. New York, NY: International Universities Press, 1971.

Groddeck, W. (1923). *Au fond de l'homme, cela.* Paris: Gallimard, 1963. [*The Book of the It.* New York, NY: Funk & Wagnalis, 1950.].

Heredia, J. M. (1900). *The Trophies (Sonnets)* (trans. F. Sewall). Kessinger Publishing, 2010.

Hinde, R. (1960). Energy models of motivation, models and analogues in biology. *Symposia of the Society of Experimental Biology*, 14: pp. 199–212. Cambridge: Cambridge University Press.

Hochmann, J., & Jeannerod, M. (1991). *Esprit où est-tu*. Paris: Odile Jacob.

Kemper, K. A. (1965). L'interprétation par allusion: Ses rapports avec les relations et les perceptions préverbales. *Revue française de psychanalyse*, 29(1): pp. 89–104.

Kestemberg, E. (2001). *La psychose froide*. Paris: Presses Universitaires de France.

Jones, E. (1957). *Sigmund Freud: Life and work. Vol. 3: The last phase, 1919–1939*. London: Hogarth.

Jones, E. (1969). *Théorie et pratique de la psychanalyse*. Paris: Payot.

Jouvet, M. (1992). *Le sommeil et le rêve*. Paris: Odile Jacob.

Laplanche, J. (1987). *New foundations for psychoanalysis* (trans. D. Macey). Oxford: Basil Blackwell, 1989.

Laplanche, J. (2007). Freud and the *sexual: Essays, 2000–2006* (trans. J. Fletcher, J. House, N. Ray). New York, NY: International Psychoanalytic Books, 2011.

Laplanche, J., & Pontalis, J. B. (1964). Fantasme originaire, fantasme des origines, origines du fantasme. *Les Temps Modernes*, 215: pp. 1833–1868.

Lubin, A. (1946). Porteurs de lances. In *Passage clandestine*. Paris: Gallimard, 2005, pp. 55–56.

Marty, P., & de M'Uzan, M. (1963). La pensée opératoire. *Revue française de psychanalyse*, 27: pp. 345–356. Republished in 1994 in *Revue française psychosomatique*, 6: pp. 197–207.

Masson, J. M. (ed.) (1985). *The complete letters of Sigmund Freud to Wilhelm Fliess, 1887–1904*. London: The Belknap Press.

McDougall, J. (2008). L'artiste et le psychanalyste. In J. André (ed.), *L'artiste et le psychanalyste*. Paris: Presses Universitaires Françaises, pp. 11–33.

Monod, J. (1970). *Le hasard et la nécessité*. Paris: Seuil.

Norton, J. (1963). Treatment of a dying patient. *Psychoanalytic Study of the Child*, 18: pp. 541–560.

Ogden, T. (1999). The analytic third: Working with intersubjective facts. *International Journal of Psychoanalysis*, 75(1): pp. 3–19.

Pantin, C. (1968). *The relations between the sciences*. Cambridge: Cambridge University Press.

Rimbaud, A. (1972). *Oeuvres completes*. Bibliothèque de la Pléiade. Paris: Gallimard.

Ritvo, L. (1992). *L'ascendant de Darwin sur Freud*. Paris: Gallimard.

Rosenfeld, I. (1988). *The invention of memory: A new view of the brain*. New York, NY: Basic Books.

Tausk, V. (1919). On the origin of the "influencing machine" in schizophrenia. *Psychoanalytic Quarterly*, 2: pp. 519–556, 1933.

Viderman, S. (1970). *Construction de l'espace analytique*. Paris: Denoël.

Winnicott, D. W. (1971). *Playing and reality*. London: Tavistock.

Index

For Product Safety Concerns and Information please contact our EU representative GPSR@taylorandfrancis.com
Taylor & Francis Verlag GmbH, Kaufingerstraße 24, 80331 München, Germany

www.ingramcontent.com/pod-product-compliance
Lightning Source LLC
LaVergne TN
LVHW021130300926
849160LV00010B/952
* 9 7 8 0 3 6 7 1 9 3 6 7 6 *